Perhaps You Misheard My Prayer?

A CANCER DETOUR ON THE PATH WITH GOD

VICKY KASEORG

ISBN-13: 978-1542520133

ISBN-10: 1542520134

Edited by Amy Fox
Cover design & Formatting by Perry Elisabeth Design
Cover painting by Vicky Kaseorg

Discovery

A lump. I was certain it was a lump, and I had never felt one there before. In a week, my daughter Asherel was getting married. How should I deal with this lump? Why now!? I felt that section of my breast again. There was no doubt.

For two nights, I did nothing but pray. I felt the lump and tried to determine if it was growing, shrinking, the same...It was probably nothing. Most lumps are benign. Cysts. Calcification. Just to be cautious, I called the diagnostic breast center where I was scheduled for a mammogram anyway in two months.

"I found a lump. Since I have a mammogram in May, I am wondering if we can just move it up and should we look at this lump?"

The nurse did not seem to think it was nothing. She took it very seriously, and wanted to move the appointment up to the following week. I told her it would have to wait another week after that. My daughter was getting married and we would be travelling to the wedding.

The mammogram was scheduled. I didn't tell my daughter about it. I didn't want to mar the wedding. And I wasn't worried. There was nothing to worry about. Each day I felt the lump to see if it was getting smaller. I tried not to think about it at all till I returned from the wedding.

The doctors were amazed I had found such a small lump in my dense breast tissue. They applauded my careful and regular self-exam. So many women don't bother with that.

The mammogram revealed a mass. The biopsy was scheduled immediately. Results came a week later. I had breast cancer.

Just like that, my life went from overly stressful to bust-major-arteries-stressful. Breast cancer? *Me?* People like me don't get breast cancer. I prefer broccoli to chocolate chip cookies. I exercise, some even say *to excess*. There is no history of breast cancer in my family.

What did I do to tick God off so terribly?

Praising God in the Midst of Struggle

March 16, 2016

Here is my cancer treatment strategy until docs take over: kayak and be happy in God's beautiful kingdom. I don't have any scientific proof, but it makes sense to me that a body overwhelmed with grief and loss is not a healing environment.

So after the diagnosis two days ago of invasive mammary carcinoma, I made a choice. I *will* praise God. I *will* choose joy. I *will* choose delight in all that I have. I *will* find laughter in the midst of fear. I *will* kayak until the surgery that may put the kibosh on kayaking for a while.

The first thing I did was cancel a haircut I had scheduled. Why spend money when my hair is going to fall out anyway? I chuckled thinking this. Then I found out I may not even need chemo, and I may retain my hair. Drat. Shouldn't have cancelled the appointment!

Friends and family poured out of every crack of my existence, calling, emailing, and texting with notes of encouragement and love, offers of help, advice, and kindness. Add to my list of happy thoughts: *I am so blessed.*

At night, in the quiet darkness is when fears have a way of nibbling away at one's hope. I found myself saying out loud, "No." *I don't want this. I don't know how to do this.* And a deep heaviness settled over me. But I have been consciously saying instead at those times, "Yes, God." *Yes* I know You are there. *Yes* I know You are with me. *Yes* I know all things work together for the good of those who know the Lord, who are called according to His purpose. *Yes* I will trust you when the darkness closes in. A calm passes over me, the dread dispels, and I feel comforted.

Today, I go for an MRI to further assess the extent of the cancer. So far, it looks like there are only two small lumps, and no lymph node involvement. This is all very good, and my "stage" is zero. That's the best stage to have if you must have cancer. I am praying the MRI confirms that initial impression.

I have done little research yet. My precious daughter-in-law and sister have done the research for me, with recommendations of surgeons and steps forward. My husband is handling all the insurance issues so I don't have to even think about it. My job: kayak and praise God.

<u>Isaiah 41:10</u>

Fear not, for I am with you; be not dismayed, for I am your God; I will strengthen you, I will help you, I will uphold you with my righteous right hand.

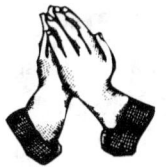

Lacing Joy in the Midst of Despair

March 17, 2016

So, yesterday I went on a run and the Bradford Pear were in full glorious bloom! So beautiful! God has given me so much to be joyful about. I could obsess about cancer, or I could smile at the billows of flowers against the Carolina blue sky. Choose to smile!

Then, after my shower, on to the MRI to see what other joys my poor body might have hidden from the impending scapel. The MRI was inconclusive, which means more biopsies (not fun)...but I did find out some good things. First, I am NOT so claustrophobic that I cannot do an MRI. Secondly, I am NOT allergic to the dye they shot into my veins to highlight whatever cancerous growths might be lurking. Thirdly, twenty minutes lying stock still while a machine whirls around you going KERPLUNK every few milliseconds affords plenty of time to pray.

I prayed for my folks, my kids, my siblings, my friends....I sang "Jesus Loves Me" (in my head) in cadence with the KERPLUNKS. I recited scripture. It was *almost* peaceful.

And there was the first piece of good news I have heard since getting the breast cancer diagnosis. I have GREAT RECEPTORS. Don't worry if you don't know what those are. I didn't either till my doc called me. I still don't *really* know what they are, but not everyone has *great* ones, and those that *do* respond really well to a critical medicine in cancer treatment. Yay me.

Here's the deal. This is a SEVERE struggle. It is not like a hangnail. It is serious. But in the midst of it, God sends little beacons of light, of joy. Bradford Pear blossoms that frame the street with breathtaking beauty. The kindness of friends giving gifts that will calm nerves; while others send healing oils for my body. The call from a breast cancer survivor with advice—cheering me on, and reminding me God is there right beside me. Having great receptors (whatever they are), and a doctor that tells me, "I want you to know I am praying for you."

No one expects joy with a cancer diagnosis. How gracious of God to lace the despair with such inexplicable moments of blessing.

2 Corinthians 4:8-9

We are afflicted in every way, but not crushed; perplexed, but not driven to despair; persecuted, but not forsaken; struck down, but not destroyed.

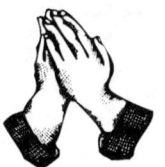

Good News in the Darkness

March 18, 2016

My little art class of young girls filed into the house. As each one entered, she said, "I am sorry for your diagnosis. I want you to know that my whole family is praying for you."

I have never felt so supported and loved. It would have been nice to feel that *without* the threat of dying hanging over my head, but it is very comforting.

It is funny how priorities change, perceptions alter, when you are faced with such a difficult illness. For example, the nurse called yesterday and her first sentence was, "Hi Mrs. K, *good news!*" What would *you* think when you hear Good News? *I won the lottery! A rich uncle I didn't know I had left me a million dollars and a horse! The biopsy was benign; we made a mistake.*

Guess what the *good news* was?

I get to have a core biopsy *today* instead of waiting a few days! *Aren't you all jealous!?* I get to go have them insert a needle (again) into my sore breast, then have them squeeze, prod, pound and smash to get the biopsy and pictures they need. Doesn't that sound fun? Good news indeed!

But it *is* good news. They moved mountains to get me in early rather than having to wait nearly two more weeks for answers. It is probably the last diagnostic procedure I will need before the surgery. And it is good news because instead of delaying things another week or more, I get to keep the meeting as scheduled with the surgeon on the 28th.

Last night, I rubbed frankincense oil on the diseased part, and prayed. The frankincense is a gift of a friend who says the biblical oils are powerful in supporting the immune system. I don't know if it was coincidence or not, but I slept the best night sleep I have had in ages. And when I awoke, I praised God for opening my eyes to the beautiful day. I washed my hands with homemade lavender soap, a gift from one of my art students. Scents of love drifted about me all night and day.

I am learning something very valuable as I deal with this cancer diagnosis. I am learning that the more my heart is centered on praising God and finding the blessings around me, the less I worry and fret. The more grateful I am for what I have already been given, and the more I remember all the wonderful moments of my life, the less fear enters my thoughts. It is hard to praise and curse simultaneously.

I may change my tune when they hack my breast off, but for now, God is a real and present comfort. And He is working through so many kind, and loving friends, family, and strangers. The real Good News is that no matter what happens to my body, my soul is secure and is bound for eternity. Good news indeed!

Revelation 21:3

And I heard a loud voice from the throne saying, "Behold, the dwelling place of God is with man. He will dwell with them, and they will be his people, and God himself will be with them as their God.

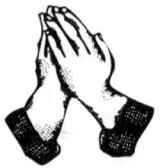

Counting It Joy

March 19, 2016

You would not think a day with a double biopsy of a very sore breast would be a blessed day. But it was! First, the doc warned me that if they could not find the suspicious mass by ultrasound guided biopsy, they would have to repeat the MRI for an MRI guided biopsy. I did not want another IV and dye which makes me feel funny, nor twenty more minutes in the coffin-like apparatus. So praise God that they found the suspicious lump on the ultrasound, biopsied it, and found another. Lather, rinse, repeat. At least I didn't need another MRI. Lucky me!

As I was leaving, feeling grateful it was over, I got a text. A friend was offering a car at a very low price to one of the mamas I work with who chose life over abortion. I volunteer as a sidewalk counselor at Charlotte's busiest abortion center. Our organization, cities4life, (charlotte.cities4life.org) has an awesome model: bring the hope of the Gospel to these desperate moms, and then meet their needs as best we can.

This particular mama wanted to leave an immoral lifestyle to follow God...but lost access to a car in the process. I was ecstatic as I connected my wonderful friend with the happy mama. See!!!! When you trust God and do what He asks, He opens the floodgates of blessing!

And then, this was almost the best part of this wonderful day. A week ago, I met "Sam" (fake name) while teaching art at the nursing home where I volunteer. Sam owns a champion Morgan stallion. But because Sam is wheelchair bound, and the drive to see the horse is too difficult and far for his wife to bring him, Sam hasn't seen the horse in a very long time.

His wife called me when the Activity Director told her what I hoped to do for Sam. I had offered to drive Sam to see his horse. I have an Occupational Therapy degree. Dealing with disabilities and wheelchairs doesn't scare me. She was so happy, and wants to come with us to see the horse. I cannot wait! Next Friday, I will drive this elderly couple to visit their champion Morgan, and I get to see Sam's face as he touches his beloved horse again. Blessings abound!

THEN, a total stranger called me to ask about my children's art classes. I told her I was happy to have her daughter join our class, but I wasn't sure how the rest of the semester would go because of my breast cancer diagnosis. This woman offered all kinds of advice. I am new to having a serious illness...but already I can tell you, *everyone has a cure*. And they all want to let you know about it. Now that is fine, and loving, and great, but it is overwhelming. I could not possibly read or do all the things people are telling me I should read or do or eat. I did gladly let her pray for me.

I never understood that line in the biblical book of James about "count it all joy when you encounter trials." Joy? In trials? Is James out of his noodle?

But now, I understand. When a trial you CANNOT get through on your own slams into you, suddenly all you have is God. And that is when God shows you, *He is enough.* I have never experienced this before. I do not want cancer, don't get me wrong, but the aura of heaven is sooo strong and so with me right now, that cancer is almost insignificant.

James 1:2-4

Count it all joy, my brothers, when you meet trials of various kinds, for you know that the testing of your faith produces steadfastness. And let steadfastness have its full effect, that you may be perfect and complete, lacking in nothing.

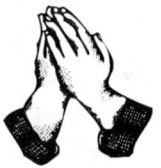

Shout Hallelujah All Day

March 20, 2016

Most cancer patients undergo chemo. It is the part I am most afraid of but it is probably inevitable. I find out when I meet with the surgeon in two Mondays. However, I found a way to conquer this fear.

First, identify it. What am I afraid of?

Feeling crappy.

Ok. Besides that?

Going bald.

Ok. And what did you ALWAYS wish you could do because you are so fickle about your hair?

Push a button and it would instantly grow. Change color. Change style. Change texture.

Well guess what??You CAN do that. Get a wig.

HMMMMMM.

So I went online researching wigs. I am here to tell you there are some VERY cute, realistic wigs out there. And who says I have to get a short grey wig to match my current mop? How about an iridescent rainbow wig with luxurious shoulder length curls? Or red? Or blonde...and discover if they really do have more fun.

Do you know what happened the more I giggled over the wigs? The less fear I felt, and the more I wanted a wig. Even if I *don't* need chemo, I may get a wig. How nice to have a clean, styled hairdo right at my fingertips when having a bad hair day.

Then, as I was still smiling over my new wig ideas, I got a gift from sister Wendy. It was a box full of trinkets, but one was exceptional—a red pendant of a horse in a beautiful silver setting. I was wearing purple, but I put the red pendant on. I didn't care if someone looked at me and wondered if I knew red and purple don't go together. It doesn't matter in the face of the reality I am encountering.

The day before I had talked with a friend who is a cancer survivor. She plans to climb Mt. Kilimanjaro this summer. She told me that chemo is hard, but I would only have a few hard days in between lots of good ones. I would still be able to walk, bike, kayak, and visit my folks. She did warn that chemo makes food taste strange, and bland food would be all I'd likely want to eat.

So, I told my husband it was time to use our gift card from my son and daughter-in-law to a fancy restaurant. We'd had the card three months. I was saving it for a special occasion. Maybe that is not a good idea. Maybe the special occasion is *today*. Let's celebrate.

So we did. I am glad there will be no cancer in heaven, but it *is* teaching me things here on earth every day.

1. If you go bald, wear a wig. Or a pretty scarf. Your scalp just became your blank canvas!

2. Wear colors that clash, and laugh at the absurd. Sometimes that is all you get to laugh at and laughter is healing.

3. Today is special. Celebrate.

My Bible study yesterday had a special verse.

> But those who want the best for me,
> Let them have the last word—a glad shout!—
> and say, over and over and over,
> "GOD is great—everything works
> together for good for his servant."
> I'll tell the world how great and good you are,
> I'll shout Hallelujah all day, every day.
> **Psalm 35:28 (The Message Translation)**

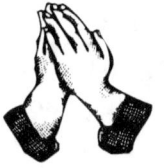

Unfamiliar Paths

March 21, 2016

I asked my art class of young girls what things they wanted to draw. Then I wrote a list with each little girl's desire, and have been ticking off the items each week in our art class. One girl is crazy about dragons. I am not really a big dragon fan, nor do I think I have EVER drawn one. However, childhood is a time for dreams coming true, and this was a simple dream I could make reality for the little girl. Another child wanted a volcano. We decided dragons and volcanoes would work well together, and the girls agreed that should be the subject for this week's class.

Dragons are not my usual fare, so I asked the girl what dragon we should draw. She gave me the name of a favorite, Nightwing. I researched Nightwing on the internet, and also found a fantasy scene that dragons might live in. Then I spent yesterday practicing the dragon in the volcano scene. This will not be easy for the girls, but with the grace of God, I think we can pull it off.

I did not expect to enjoy drawing dragons as much as I did. Had the little girl not asked for it, I might have spent my *entire life* as an artist never drawing a dragon. I considered this in light of the path God is currently leading me. Choosing *on my own* to be diagnosed with breast cancer, and face the rather daunting prospects before me for the next year would *never* have happened.

However, having little choice, I am embarking on this path. In the process, I am discovering many of the same truths I discovered complying with the little girl's suggestion that we draw a dragon.

1. If you have learned to trust God in the small things, you have all you need to trust God in the harder things. In fact, in some ways it is easier to trust God in the hard things because you have NO DOUBT you *cannot* do it on your own power.

2. When taking a path you would never have taken on your own, you learn you can do things you never thought you would, or could do. Sometimes being forced to walk a road you would rather not walk is the only way to learn you CAN.

3. Every new step taken in faith brings unexpected blessings. The less familiar the path you are urged to travel, the greater the trust required, and the greater assurance you are guided by something greater than yourself.

4. There is immense contentment and joy that you submitted to *His* will, not your will, because the promise of what awaits at the completion is so glorious.

Unfamiliar paths are frightening. For example, I was terrified when I began volunteering as a sidewalk counselor at the abortion center. Yet, as more and more women turned to Christ and chose life because we were there to speak for their babies, it became my favorite activity! In fact, I go there this morning as I do every Monday.

I liked how my dragon turned out. I can't wait to guide the little girls in drawing one themselves!

Isaiah 42:16

I will lead the blind by ways they have not known, along unfamiliar paths I will guide them; I will turn the darkness into light before them and make the rough places smooth. These are the things I will do; I will not forsake them.

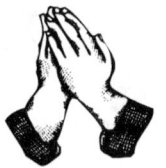

Chemo Has its Perks

March 23, 2016

The bad news is the second set of biopsies of two more lumps found by the very thorough team at CMC showed another cancerous lump. One was benign, but now with three malignant lumps, my guess is my breast is going the way of the dinosaur. When the nurse called me, I was at the vet with Lucky for his annual check-up. I couldn't talk or ask questions. When I sat in the car, a flood of tears threatened. Instead, I asked God to take my fear and sadness away. Lucky looked at me. The despair subsided.

Chemo is probably in my future. I find out for sure Monday when I meet with the surgeon, but I am a realist. Fortunately, I am a realist with an abiding faith in God. He has supernaturally kept me calm, and even joyful. Please do not misunderstand. If I didn't have to have cancer, I would definitely not be picking it to go with my Easter dress. However, God has a plan, and I trust it is a good one. I can mourn and cry and scream and rage...and probably will on low days....but it does no good. It is what it is. May as well have fun with it....

So, I went wig shopping. I met one of the nicest human beings on earth in Gastonia, NC. Her name is Ginny, and she owns Ginny's Wigs. (www.ginnyswigs.com) I called to warn her that I was coming. I explained I was not ready to buy until the surgeon told me I would be getting chemo, and I would be losing my hair. However, I wanted to look at wigs now. She told me to come on down!

As I drove over, I wondered if I would cry. My hair is important to me. I don't even know why it is SO important. It shouldn't be. It *is* pretty nice hair. Thick. Easy to style. Grey. I never colored it because I thought one should accept whatever God gives.

Ginny had other ideas.

"Try this," she said. It was not grey.

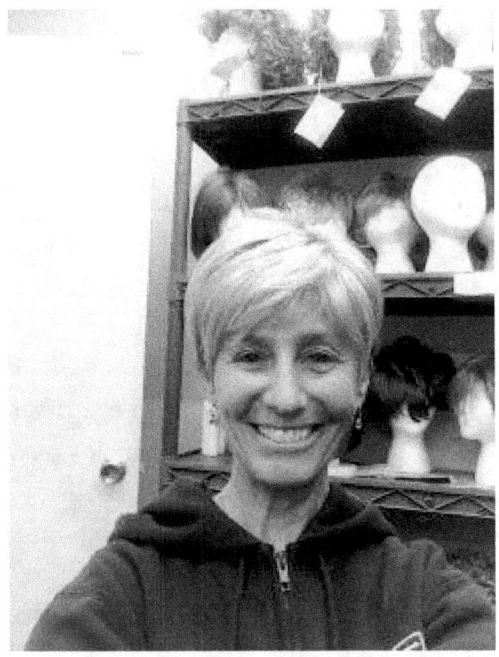

Hmmm. I have to admit, blonde takes ten...maybe twenty years off of me.

"Now *this* is a really cute wig," Ginny said.

I agreed! It was very cute!

"Or, a little less blonde...." Ginny handed me another one.

Even cuter!

Hmmmm. I am beginning to think cancer is not so bad....

Then I asked Ginny about how these wigs hold up to running, kayaking, biking....If at ALL possible, I am not giving up those things.

Ginny considered this problem. Well, in all honesty, lots of perspiration would indeed decrease the life of the wig. So, here is a fun solution. When I exercise, I wear a wig *hat* and get instant long hair! I can even pull it back in a ponytail. The hat is a regular hat. The hair sticks out from the bottom, but only is attached to the bottom fifth of the hat. Much cooler than a wig, and the perspiration only goes on the hat. Which is washable. Problem solved.

Ginny and I were having a great time. I didn't feel at all like crying. I was having a blast seeing what I looked like as a blond. To tell you the truth, I looked much less like an old hag. I should have gotten cancer ten years ago!

The whole time I was there, I was eying the purple wig. My daughter recently dyed her hair purple. I kind of like it.

"Could I try on the purple wig?" I asked Ginny. Not because I would really buy it. I won't. But because laughter is restorative, and I knew it would make me laugh.

I was right. It did. It made us both laugh.

See. God is good. *He is present wherever you look when you are certain that wherever you look, He is there.* Ginny started her business because she felt bad for those she knew who suffered hair loss. And then one day she realized she had a booming business. That isn't what drives her though. It is the smiles of women facing devastating illness who she makes beautiful in the midst of such trauma.

If I had a million dollars, I would get the purple wig too.

<u>James 1:2-4</u>

Count it all joy, my brothers, when you meet trials of various kinds,
for you know that the testing of your faith produces steadfastness.
And let steadfastness have its full effect, that you may be perfect and
complete, lacking in nothing.

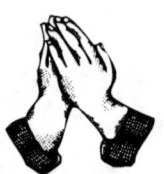

Lessons From the Wind

March 24, 2016

Little did I know that the wind was determined to teach me yet another lesson about hardships. As if a cancer diagnosis was not chock full of enough lessons to last me for the next...oh, lifetime or *two*...God sent the wind to reveal His truth yesterday.

Knowing that once the surgery is done, I will be sidelined at least two weeks or so, I am using every moment I can to kayak. So I dashed off to my favorite lake. As soon as I arrived, I knew I was in trouble. My hat was nearly blown off my head. I realized if I were wearing a wig, which I would be after chemo, it would be blown to the next county by this wind.

So while unloading my kayak (despite my inner voice saying ARE YOU NUTS???? YOU CAN'T KAYAK IN THIS WIND!!!!) I began to muse over sister Amy's suggestion that I stencil hair on my bald head. The pictures on the internet of bald heads with stenciled hair are lovely...but mostly because the models are knock-you-down gorgeous with expertly applied makeup and taut unwrinkled skin. Face it, the stencils would not have the same effect on me. (When my head is is bald. It isn't yet.)

Back to the task at hand. I launched, and was quickly wondering if the beauty of the lake was worth the shellacking I was going to receive at the hand of the wind. It was brutal. The gusts had to be 30 mph or more. There were times I was paddling as hard as I could, and not moving.

Then my doctor's office called. Here is a tasty tidbit for those of you about to embark on a new cancer adventure. Every day some medical person is calling for one reason or another. I answered my cell phone, and was quickly blown downwind to the far end of the lake at a pretty *spectacular* pace.

Normally, I can kayak that distance back to where I started in no time. Not against a hurricane, however. I ended the phone call, and began the extremely arduous journey back to the dock. I looked in the *distant* distance at the dock, paddling for all I was worth. I did not appear to be gaining an inch.

So I changed my focus. I only looked at the trough of the wave in front of me. *Just make it to the next trough, crest the wind tossed wave, and then focus on the trough after that.*

Slowly, straining with all my might, I made it from trough to trough. Sometimes the wind would die down a little, and I paddled furiously to gain as much ground as possible before it roared to full throttle again. In this manner, I advanced.

And understood.

When we face a daunting trial for the foreseeable future, looking all the way to the end of the road we will travel is usually discouraging. Better to look straight ahead at only the next step. And then focus on the one after that. There may be lots of lows, the troughs of life. Only take one at a time. Take advantage of the lulls in between the really hard parts, but don't try to anticipate *all* the hard parts to determine if you have the strength.

You don't. None of us do.

But God does. It is very merciful that God rarely reveals more than one step at a time. He only gave one day of manna at a time to His people as they wandered through the desert for forty years. He reminds us we are only to consider the troubles of today. It will have enough to occupy us, and tomorrow's troubles should not be borrowed in advance. It's not like there is such a shortage of troubles that we should hoard them ahead of time.

Such good advice. Thank you, Wind.

I made my way slowly, but steadily. In half an hour, I reached the dock. I was so amazed at how I had successfully battled that terrible wind, that I decided to keep going past the dock, against the wind until I was *totally* tired. I was only 3/4ths tired thus far. I would not have to work at all to return to the dock. The wind would blow me effortlessly home.

When my arms began to ache and my reserves were depleted, I turned the kayak around. With the wind now blessedly at my back, I stopped paddling. The wind carried me on angel's wings back to the dock. Since no one else was foolish enough to be out in that wind, I made up a song and sang it out loud. It was about how God will carry me safely home. It was not Grammy-worthy, but only me and the wind heard it anyway.

Ephesians 4:14

So that we may no longer be children, tossed to and fro by the waves and carried about by every wind of doctrine, by human cunning, by craftiness in deceitful schemes.

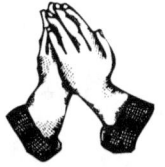

God Has Me in His Sights

March 25, 2016

I got a text from one of the Moms I work with who recently chose life for her baby rather than abortion.

"Don't forget to send me my daily Bible verse."

Music to my ears!

"I won't. I have been sending you one every day. Have you checked your email?"

"OH! I will right now."

Later I talked with her and she told me that she is overwhelmed. Not with the baby. There is no doubt in her mind that God would have her keep the baby. Just with life, school, struggles...

"I really need to be reading those Bible verses you send," she told me, "They help keep me positive."

Don't I know it!!! I told her not to be afraid to ask us if there was anything we could do to help in specific needs. We can't *always* help, and we make no promises, but we will try.

"I want to get my associate degree...but I have to take classes online. I need a computer. Used, not fancy...but I can't do it without a computer. I'm not complaining," she told me, "Everyone has troubles. I am reading my Bible and trying to stay strong."

"I hear you," I said, relating more than ever with my recent cancer diagnosis.

As soon as I got off the phone, I texted her a Bible verse so she didn't have to check her email.

Then I checked my own mail. Real mail. I went to the mailbox. There was a mystery box from Amazon. I didn't order anything. What was it??

It was a book by one of my favorite authors, Bill Bryson. Bryson always makes me laugh. I know my sisters understand I intend to laugh my way to health. I suspect one of them sent it, but there was no note to clue me as to the sender. I guessed right, when I emailed the one I thought had this gift written all over her. Notes and emails and texts of encouragement and prayer have been pouring in as well. I am blessed.

I know God has me, and the mama who is overwhelmed in His sights, but it is so encouraging to know fellow humans do too.

<u>Genesis 41:52</u>
God has made me fruitful in the land of my misfortunes.

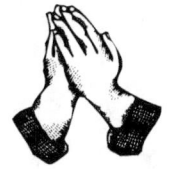

Lessons from a Horse

March 27, 2016

In just one more day, I find out what the surgeon plans to do to my cancerous breast. I'm still praying for a miracle, but short of that, praying for peace in the midst of whatever I will be facing. Meanwhile, I am continuing *life,* doing what brings me joy. To that end, I had a special day planned for Good Friday.

Remember, I met "Sam" a couple of months ago at the nursing home where I teach art. Soon, somehow we were discussing our mutual love of horses and he showed me pictures on his phone of his beautiful Morgan horse. Sam had not seen the horse in four months because of the logistics of the long drive, being wheelchair bound, and his wife having had surgery recently. Neither he nor his wife, "Elle", were up to driving themselves, but both missed their horse terribly.

When I heard this, I knew what my *happiness medicine* for the week would be. Take Sam and Elle to see their horse. I arranged the details with Elle, and we set Friday for our trip to see the horse. Despite predictions of thunderstorms that would have cancelled our trip, the day dawned clear without a storm in sight. That was God's first anointing of our plans.

I could not wait! As we drove, I got to hear the incredible history of this amazing couple. For their privacy, I will not share it with you, but I was enthralled. Delightful, accomplished people, but best of all, the tender kindness with which they treated each other. The long drive went by in an instant.

And then, we pulled into the farm, and Sam saw his horse. He rolled down his window and called to the horse, who came to the fence right away. It took us a little huffing, puffing, and some shaky moments on uneven ground, but we managed to get Sam safely in the wheelchair, and then onto the pasture.

Here is a picture of him greeting his horse for the first time in four months.

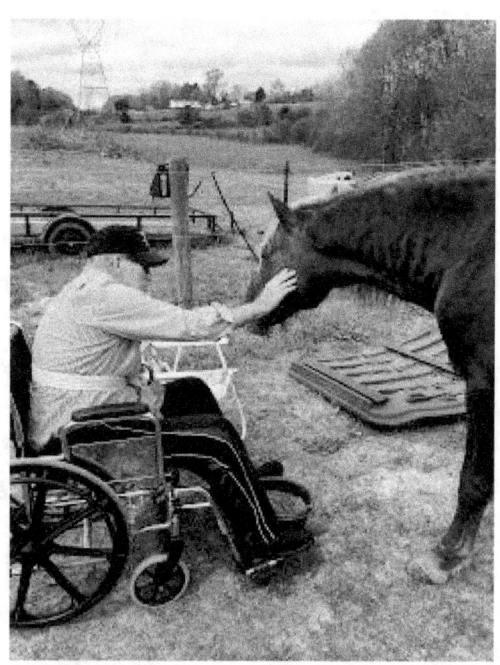

Kind of makes you want to cry, doesn't it? We communed with the horse for two hours. We had packed a picnic lunch, and sat in the sunshine eating our lunch while the horse munched his hay. I can't remember the last time I enjoyed two hours so completely.

After I dropped the grateful couple back at the nursing home, I thought about how hard it is to grow old, to face illness, to face limitations, and ultimately, mortality. What we know and love will pass away. That is a certainty. Some of us fight this truth with bitterness and anger. We refuse to accept the hand we have been dealt, and forget that *everything* we are given is an unearned blessing.

Charles Spurgeon noted that God could crush us, and certainly *should*, were we to receive what our sin deserves. Instead, *"There," said He, "that self-same arm which made thee quake, see there, I give it to thee. Go out and live. I have made thee mighty as I am, to do My works; I will put strength into thee. The same strength which would have broken thee to pieces on the wheel shall now be put into thee, that you may do mighty works."*

In spite of all the terrors and traps of our mortal world, God strengthens us to *go out and live*. Live in His might, with His strength, so that we may do mighty works.

Easter Sunday is here. The supreme example of sacrificial love is exemplified and fulfilled in this special day. Jesus knew the agony that awaited Him on the cross, and asked God that if it be possible, the cup He was about to drink would pass Him by. YET, and on this YET the full message of submission to God lies, "Yet not as *I* will, but as *you* will."

Go out and live. Rejoice in the soft muzzle of a horse in your palm. Enjoy what God has given. Help others. Cradle joy in your heart in simple pleasures knowing none of it is permanent. Live in submission to His will, and the victory is won. He is risen.

At least, I think that is what God was whispering in the quiet peace of the pasture.

John 6:37-39

[37] All those the Father gives me will come to me, and whoever comes to me I will never drive away. [38] For I have come down from heaven not to do my will but to do the will of him who sent me. [39] And this is the will of him who sent me, that I shall lose none of all those he has given me, but raise them up at the last day.

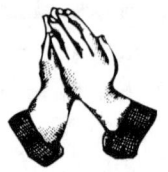

I Should Rejoice

March 28, 2016

I don't always feel the way I *should* feel. I should praise the Lord that I have awoken to a new day. I should notice the vibrant colors around me, the warmth of the sun, the sound of the birds. I should praise God that I have the strength to lift my arms, open my eyes, stand on my own two feet. I should rejoice each moment that God saw fit to miraculously meld perfect justice and perfect mercy in the atoning death and resurrection of Jesus for my sins. I should dance every morning in the glowing promise of eternal life.

This morning, I head off to the sidewalks of the abortion center to encourage abortion-minded mamas to choose life instead for their babies. Every Monday, this is my privilege and mission. It has a special poignancy for me since my cancer diagnosis. It is an interesting juxtaposition: counseling those who would so casually discard life while I so desperately cling to it. I have little doubt that Satan wants the cancer to stop me from coming here. It makes me want to come here *all the more*, since I see with even sharper clarity the precious gift of life.

As soon as I am done at the sidewalk, I meet for the first time with the oncology surgeon. I will get my first official diagnosis, clear understanding of what I am facing, and treatment plan. I want to be like the person in the picture I described in my opening paragraph, but to be truthful, yesterday I was scared, and sad. It does not promise to be a fun journey for the next few months.

I read more about alternative cancer treatments, holistic health, and how to promote the immune system. I find them more and more compelling. I have already started some of the simple suggestions. Frankincense oil rubbed on the area of tumors, baking soda/lemon water several times a day to increase alkalinity of the body (cancer cells apparently don't thrive in an alkaline environment,) bone broth soup. Long walks. Happy thoughts. Lots of prayer.

I already eat really healthily, but I have added even more healthy fare to my larder. Hummus and broccoli for snacks, leafy greens, yogurt and blueberries...

I know my friend Carolyn would add icky things like liver and chicken feet, but I draw the line on those.

For almost a month now, I have lived with the knowledge of this awful disease lurking inside me. I have been supernaturally sustained, cheerful and upbeat. My cancer survivor friend warned me: *there will be bad days. Days when you struggle. Give yourself freedom to accept that. It does not show lack of faith because you have down days. There will be many lessons on this journey, but sometimes you won't see anything worthwhile...just that it stinks.*

God gives us a similar message in Psalm 38. The psalmist (David) cries out to God in weary distress: (v.9-10)

All my longings lie open before you, Lord;
my sighing is not hidden from you.
My heart pounds, my strength fails me; even the light has gone from my eyes.
(v. 17) For I am about to fall,
and my pain is ever with me.
(v. 21-22) LORD, *do not forsake me;*
do not be far from me, my God
Come quickly to help me,
my Lord and my Savior.

Wow! Can I relate! Poor David ends the psalm without a solution, only his anguished despair, and recognition that his life is in God's hands. We should face life with a hopeful joy before God, but sometimes, it is just plain too exhausting to keep the mournful thoughts at bay.

Fortunately, those periods are not permanent. Look at Psalm 40: 1-4, my reading for today:

> *I waited patiently for the L*ORD*;*
>> *he turned to me and heard my cry.*
> *² He lifted me out of the slimy pit,*
>> *out of the mud and mire;*
> *he set my feet on a rock*
>> *and gave me a firm place to stand.*
> *³ He put a new song in my mouth,*
>> *a hymn of praise to our God.*
> *Many will see and fear the L*ORD
>> *and put their trust in him.*
> *⁴ Blessed is the one*
>> *who trusts in the L*ORD*,*
> *who does not look to the proud,*
>> *to those who turn aside to false gods*

What a contrast from David's lament just two psalms earlier! God WILL lift me out of the slimy pit. He will lift *all* of us out. All we have to do is put our trust in Him. Around midnight last night, suddenly I felt a lifting of the gloom. I felt the urge to stretch out my arms, palms up to the ceiling. Inexplicable comfort and joy flooded through me. The air seemed gentle, softer.

Someone must be praying for me.

Whoever it was, thank you.

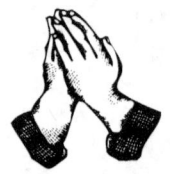

He Never Works the Way I Expect

March 29, 2016

First, HUGE praise. I went for my first consult with the oncology surgeon after my time on the sidewalk of the abortion mill counseling women to choose life. My oncologist THINKS MAYBE we can do just a lumpectomy and MAYBE no chemo if my lymph nodes are clear (He won't know that till they biopsy the lymph nodes during surgery). I have to do one more biopsy (*Big sigh*) to see if one last suspicious area is clean. If it is, he thinks we can go for lumpectomy, not full mastectomy. Oh friends, please keep praying. This is by far my preference! And no chemo maybe!!! Now, I did have some AWFULLY cute wigs already picked out, but I can live without them. I had put aside all hope for a less invasive surgery. God is opening a window....

Meanwhile, my morning at the abortion center sidewalk was amazing, and demonstrates, again, the fallacy of "pro-choice." One woman pulled into the parking lot of the abortion center already crying. She and her friend got out of the car, now both crying.

I was on the microphone, putting our sound system to good use. As an aside, the abortion center applies for the sound system every week. Only one permit is granted. The abortion center never USES a sound system, but they apply for the one permit every day as well. They just don't want us to have it because it helps CHANGE MINDS and the center loses money for every baby who lives. Mamas throughout the center can hear us when we speak over our sound system.

This week, we had the sound system. I told the mama she didn't need to do this, and if she felt this bad already, she could not imagine the pain she would feel later if she aborted. She sobbed, hugging her friend who was also crying. They stood in clear sight at the back of the car, hugging and crying for a long time. Meanwhile, I spoke nonstop to her on the microphone. I told her we could help and reminded her of God's love and provision and strength when we have reached the end of ours. (Thank you Cancer, for making me talk so knowledgeably about this particular truth.) I talked about how our circumstances should *never* dictate our moral choices.

When I was quiet, fellow counselor Chrissy spoke. We took turns speaking without pause as though a life depended on it...because it *did*. Then the "pro-choice" security escort, so noble and gentle-hearted (*Sarcasm Alert*), put her arm around the crying woman and pulled her towards the clinic. I could not hear what she was saying but I had a good guess. She was dragging the poor sobbing woman to the clinic door. The two crying women stopped and now stood in front of the car where we couldn't see them as easily. The security escort was still talking to them.

Over the mic, I advised them to listen carefully and compare the words and motivations of the escort urging the mama to abort, with our message of God and hope.

"They claim to be pro-choice, but what options are they offering you? One. Pro-death. She is telling you not to listen to our options." (It turns out, I was spot-on in my guess of what the escort was saying.)

The crying mama went in despite our pleas, and the crying friend drove away. She stopped for me in the driveway on her way out. She was sobbing. She told me she knew abortion was wrong but didn't know what else to do for her friend. I gave her my phone number and our literature and told her to go back in to her friend. Show her the literature. Tell her to call me.

She drove away, but returned a short time later, talking on the phone as she pulled into the lot. Then she pulled up to the door of the clinic and the mama came out! I called to her friend, "Will she come on our ultrasound RV???" I almost collapsed when she nodded.

She drove to the curb next to the RV and parked. The mama was sobbing, telling me she didn't know what to do. I assured her we would help her, and God was with her. I then led the broken woman (C) onto our mobile ultrasound RV along with several young kids who were the progeny of her and the friend.

They were sweet kids and sat quietly as I counseled C. After sharing the Gospel, C told me she had asked Jesus into her life the night before! She had told God then that if abortion was not the answer, could He give her a sign?

"*You* were the sign," she said. "When you kept talking on the mic, I was asking myself *why is she doing this to me?* But God was showing me what to do, and I kept hearing your voice over that security lady."

I put my art degree to good use drawing animals to keep the kids entertained while counseling C. Their dog had just been hit and killed by a car, so I asked them to describe the dog, and I drew a picture of him. They really liked that. Meanwhile, C had made her decision even before seeing the baby on the ultrasound. *No matter what,* she would follow God. She would find a way to raise this baby, or, if need be, place him for adoption. She would not kill him.

She told me that the escort was trying to talk her into aborting. "Just go in the clinic to do it. Ignore them," the escort had said, pointing at me and Chrissy. But C told me she kept hearing me say, "You don't have to do this."

When she had gone into the clinic, she'd asked if the baby's heart was already beating. She was several weeks along. She told them she would not abort if the baby's heart was beating. They told her *"NO, the heart is not beating."* What a bunch of liars!!!! The baby's heart beats at 18 days after conception, before most women even know they are pregnant!

Anyway, now safe in our RV, C and her friend were beside themselves with gratitude and even joy. The ultrasound tech, Kelly, was great. Here is God's wonderful icing on the cake: as soon as Kelly put the ultrasound on C's tummy, the baby popped into view with such an OBVIOUS heartbeat that all those little kids who were with us said, "AWWWWWWWW!" Every one of those kids, age 4-9 could tell that was a beating heart. The littlest girl told me, "That's a baby!"

Not two minutes after they drove away, I got a text from C, "THANK YOU FOR PREVENTING THE BIGGEST MISTAKE OF MY LIFE. I FEEL A LOT BETTER NOW AND STRONGER THAN EVER. I WILL FOREVER APPRECIATE YOU. I AM REALLY BLESSED TO BE ABLE TO OPEN MY EYES. I LOVE Y'ALL SO MUCH."

Get this, she wants to be an ultrasound tech, wants to go to school for it, and needs a computer. I had put out a Facebook plea for a computer for another mom I work with, and had gotten two responses! I had an extra computer for C! She was thrilled. God is SOOOOOOOOOOOOOOO good!

He never really works the way I expect, but He is ALWAYS working.

Romans 8:24-25

For in this hope we were saved. Now hope that is seen is not hope. For who hopes for what he sees? But if we hope for what we do not see, we wait for it with patience.

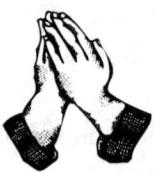

The Blessings of Cancer

March 30, 2016

I am praying for the least invasive lumpectomy for my cancer, but still preparing for whatever the new test results throw at me. Thus, I sat down and read cover to cover the very thick binder of information Levine Cancer Institute provided: *Everything You Always Wanted to Know About Breast Cancer...And Then Some*. (This is not the actual title, but should be.)

I learned many things. For one thing, breast reconstruction can be done using the patient's own fat. The most popular region to take the fat from is the tummy. The patient gets the double bonus of perky new breasts, and a tummy tuck, all for the price of one surgery!

However, the surgeon looked at me and said he didn't think I had enough tummy to do this. This is one situation where being a little chubby would have been useful. My reading revealed that there are other regions they can take fat from...like the lower buttocks. Now my lower buttocks are not very fatty...but my upper thighs are! I am petitioning the surgeon if a mastectomy is required, we do a thigh liposuction! Win/win! Just because it is usually not done this way doesn't mean it *can't* be. I am willing to be a trendsetter here if it means I get sleek thighs in the bargain.

I am also wondering if they can clean my teeth while I am under the anesthesia. I hate my bi-yearly cleaning because I have very sensitive teeth. And since they insist next year I need another colonoscopy, could they throw that in as well? As long as I am out like a light, I want all the unpleasant things in store for me to be completed in one fell swoop.

Sure, the operating room might get a little crowded, but it will be a chance for a real multi-disciplinary approach to treatment. All the doctors insist that improves patient care...They can all gather around my unconscious body and fix me to perfection then and there! (A God image if ever I saw one...)

Today, I go off for genetic testing. If I have the "cancer gene", that is a game changer. Likely looking at a double mastectomy in that case. This is ok if they are willing to rebuild both breasts using my thighs. I was called "thunder thighs" in Middle School, and have never lived it down. Maybe cancer is not a tragedy, but an *opportunity*!

I read on. I found yet another unexpected blessing from cancer. If I have the mastectomy, I am not allowed to vacuum for 6-8 weeks! Woohoo! It just keeps getting better.

Now understand, I don't want a mastectomy. However, I need to be prepared. The radiologist called yesterday expressing the issues that make me a difficult lumpectomy case. She agrees I should "give it the old college try," but I have been forewarned that it may not work out as I hope. I may have to do the mastectomy.

I am living proof that God can calm one's fears, and even give inexplicable joy in the midst of severe hardship and trials. I do not yet count it ALL joy when I encounter trials...as James in the Bible suggests. But I am seeing SOME joy...and that is major.

If circumstances determine our joy or our moral choices, then we are likely to be miserable, despicable, conscience-less creatures. One of the hardest but most freeing lessons in a faith-filled life is that real joy has nothing to do with circumstances and everything to do with our relationship with God. I suppose one of the supreme benefits of cancer, or any deep struggle, is we find out just how strong that relationship really is.

Romans 12:12

Rejoice in hope, be patient in tribulation, be constant in prayer.

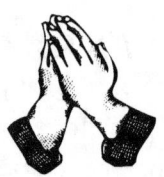

If It Weren't For Cancer, This Would Be a Vacation

March 31, 2016

I was all alone in the waiting room of the genetic testing department. I was the ONLY one there. They offered me CHAI tea. I was surrounded by quiet, mellow-hued walls, soothing plants, and the distant sound of water trickling in a decorative fountain. I felt like I was in a spa.

The cancer centers know just how to do it up right. I settled into my comfy chair, sipping my Chai tea, and thought, "If it weren't for the cancer part of this whole experience, I would think I was on an expensive vacation."

The genetic counseling was fun. They seemed very concerned that I be prepared for whatever my blood might reveal. I told them I am fine if my blood reveals I need a double mastectomy, as long as they take the fat from my thighs for the reconstruction. They patted me gently on my shoulder and thought I was joking.

Now the next unexpected blessing of the Cancer Center is that parking is free! They stamp my little parking ticket, and I could hang out there all day if I wanted to at NO COST. What fun! Who *doesn't* get a kick out of watching people hobble out of chemo, or stumble with gauze and bandages covering their face from the one-day surgery room?

Surprisingly, I found an even better way to capitalize on my free parking. Right next to the Cancer Center is the Little Sugar Creek Greenway. This greenway is the result of a project that put into practice one of my favorite philosophies of life. *Take the ugliest part of something, and make it beautiful.* So Charlotte took the polluted, trash-strewn, filthy Little Sugar Creek, and built a stunning pathway alongside it. They cleaned the creek, built parks, and erected statues and fountains along the walkway. Gorgeous pedestrian bridges were installed. Commemorative plaques and educational displays were strategically placed all along the many miles of the new greenway.

Since parking was free, I went on a long walk on the lovely greenway.

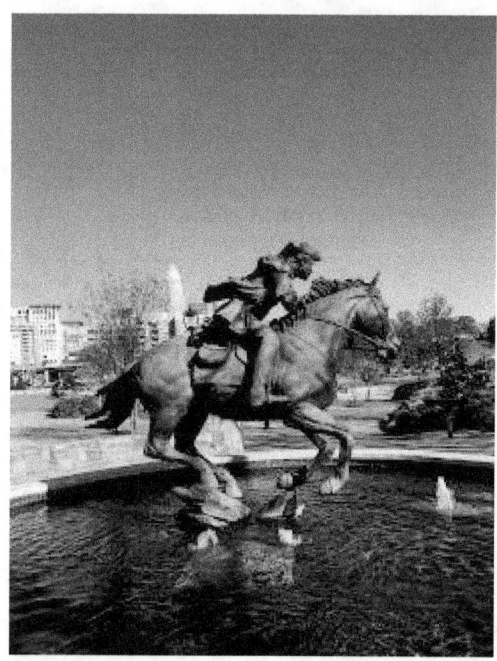

This is a magnificent statue of "Captain Jack", a patriot who rode to the Continental Congress in Philly to express Charlotte's resolve to stand with those who declared freedom from Britain. I think I have remembered that correctly. I loved the statue, and walked slowly all around it, stumped by the engineering. This is a heavy bronze statue...the weight of which is supported on three small points of contact. This does not seem possible.

That got me thinking. The weight of the world is on our shoulders. If you can't relate, give yourself time. One day you will. Everyone eventually experiences crushing burdens they cannot possibly sustain. Then, God tells us, *Trust me. I have this covered. I can bear your burden. I can hold you up and all that terrible weight with three small points of contact: the Father, the Son, and the Holy Spirit.*

I circled Captain Jack, and noticed from a picture on a plaque that the artist who made that lovely statue was very young. How could he have known at such a young age those three contact points were enough? It's taken me nearly sixty years to realize that.

John 14:26

But the Helper, the Holy Spirit, whom the Father will send in my name, he will teach you all things and bring to your remembrance all that I have said to you.

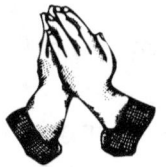

From Where Our Positive Attitude Should Arise

April 1, 2016

A whole bunch of the moms I work with who chose life over abortion are in deep crisis right now. Troubles seem to coalesce like pools of algae in a stagnant pond. I wonder why that is.

One of them called with deep struggles and the need for immediate help while I was at the plastic surgeon discussing which form of lopping off my breast would be preferable in the treatment of my cancer. I told the young lady, J, that I would call her after my doc appointment.

The plastic surgeon agreed that if I end up with a full mastectomy, and want to use my own fat tissue to reconstruct the breast, I cannot use my tummy or my thighs. Too small. (Wish I could tell those middle school bullies who used to call me "thunder thighs.") However, he said he *could* find enough fat on my buttocks to use. *Real charmer, that man.*

He said that the problem in using butt fat as the lard of choice is that it requires a ten-hour operation and five days in the hospital. Nice as it would be to get a trim bottom (which until yesterday I thought I had), it is probably not worth the trauma. Basically, we are at the same place of leaving it up to me with no really *fun* choice available. It's like being asked if you would like to have someone pull off your toenails one by one, or stick dull knives in your belly till you bleed to death. No one is offering a third option of an all-expense-paid trip to Europe to combat this disease.

I did find out that whether I get a lumpectomy or a mastectomy, I will have two operations. I hadn't known that and was not doing cartwheels upon hearing this news. First I find out I have a fat bottom, and now I find out I go under the knife *twice*, no matter what. However, if I get the mastectomy, I might need no chemo OR radiation. If I get the lumpectomy, I must go through radiation. Choices, choices!

If I get the mastectomy, there is a different method of breast reconstruction which involves basically placing a balloon inside the chest muscle at the time of surgery. Then over a period of 3 or 4 visits (*maybe less*, says the charming plastic surgeon looking at my breasts....), they blow the breasts up to the proper size. The muscle has to stretch, which is why they can't do it all at once. Then there is a second surgery to remove the temporary expander and replace with a semi-permanent one. In ten to fifteen years, that expander needs to be surgically replaced again. That is not a big deal, the surgeon told me. Easy for *him* to say.

He explained the shape is a little different...more rounded.

"Yes, I know," I said, "I've seen the movie stars."

"Right, they have had implants."

"So I will look like a movie star...but without her salary?"

"Correct."

With all this cheery new info to digest, I called the mom in crisis. I can't share details, but it involved me driving immediately across town to assist her. All is well (sort of) and it was nice to see her very pregnant belly. Life may be crumbling about me in little pieces, but that baby safely growing made me happy.

The boyfriend of the mom told me that despite their struggles, they had a positive attitude. That solves almost everything, he said. A positive attitude is certainly good, and we should all seek to maintain one, however a positive attitude based on our own strength and capabilities will definitely erode. Eventually, we will have to face the fact that we are not up to the desperate challenges of life. On the other hand, a positive attitude based on the promises of God will always sustain us. Our bodies and our minds will fail us, but God never will. He alone has overcome death, and He alone is where our hopes and positive attitude should emanate from.

<u>Joshua 1:9</u>

Have I not commanded you? Be strong and courageous. Do not be frightened, and do not be dismayed, for the Lord your God is with you wherever you go."

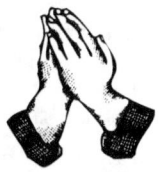

Who Needs Chemo for Hair Loss?

April 2, 2016

For eight weeks, I have needed a haircut as my normally short hair was getting straggly and difficult to style. However, I held off. I still don't know if I will need chemo for my breast cancer since all the tests are not completed. Besides that, they are waiting on other test results, thus at least another three weeks before surgery scheduled. So despite knowing that if I must undergo chemo I will lose my hair, I went to a new hairdresser for a "pixie" cut. I didn't think I could stand another month or so of my increasingly unruly hair.

My old hairdresser is on maternity leave, so I went to a new one. She was very good, but I must say, cut my hair **much** shorter than I would like. Oh well. It will grow. Unless I get chemo...in which case it will all fall out. Some dangly earrings and a pretty dress -- I bet *then* I will look like a girl.

Anyway, as long as I was out, I decided to drive to the local post-mastectomy shop. *How fun is that!* I thought it would be valuable to look at breast prostheses, mastectomy bras, swimsuits, and post-surgical camisoles. Demystifying this whole new world is important. I walked into a largely deserted, quaint boutique, and was met by a lovely, kind woman. I explained why I was there, and she took me immediately under-wing.

She showed me what sorts of things I would need if I got a lumpectomy, and what I would need with a mastectomy. I even got to heft a 38 D breast implant, and thanked God I am a small woman. It would be an aerobic workout just hauling those babies around all day.

The camisoles are designed to hold padding as needed, as well as the drainage tubes post surgery. They are NOT cheap. $75. Now I haven't talked about drainage tubes yet because of ostrich-head-in-the-sand syndrome. The drainage tubes sound like one of the yuckiest parts of this journey.

However, I felt it was time to slay this monster too. I asked her to tell me about the drainage tubes and exactly how one went about dealing with three or four tubes hanging out of your chest with stomach-churning gunk dripping out of them. She agreed this part was not fun, but brief. Two weeks for most women. They must always be pinned to the shirt or in a special camisole pocket so they don't get pulled upon. Every few hours, the patient dumps them out after measuring the output. Doesn't that sound appetizing? Hope you aren't reading this while eating.

The mastectomy bathing suits were super cute. They were the price of any good bathing suit. I found a few I liked immediately. The nice saleswoman wrote me a list with codes for insurance of all I would need with either surgical scenario. As I turned to leave, she asked if she could hug me. She seemed to be genuinely concerned for my welfare, and told me she'd be praying for me.

Driving away, I called my "nurse navigator" to ask if I could get camisoles more cheaply on-line. I could, but she told me I should visit the *Charlotte Breast Friends* in the pink house nearby. They often received donated camisoles and would give them to me free! She told me it is also a great resource with free classes and seminars for survivors.

So, I drove there, mostly because *Breast Friends* is about the cutest name for such an agency that I have ever heard. And a free $75 camisole is nothing to sneeze at.

Breast Friends is in a historic gorgeous home and as soon as you walk in, you are enveloped in hope and kindness. The volunteer, Krista, offered a tour, and told me she'd be happy to give me some camisoles. She also wanted to tell me about all the other completely free services this great ministry offers.

That sounded wonderful, but first I needed to use the restroom. Listen to this: there were hand-painted pink butterflies on the wall. Everything in this building is soothing and gentle. She invited me to a seminar coming up, which starts with a wine and food social time. I can't say cancer is the *best* thing that ever happened to me, but it has its perks.

She chose two lovely camisoles that were as soft as butter, and looked nearly new. While picking out the camisoles, she and several others in the office shared their own cancer stories and answered my questions. Every employee there was a cancer survivor and chose to use their lives to help other cancer survivors. I was so glad I had decided to stop by.

Before I left, Krista gave me a bag of goodies, including 'chemo' slippers. If I do get chemo, my feet would get cold in the chemo room. Not with those cute pink, skid-free slippers though.

"Please come back soon," Krista asked. I didn't even have to *prove* I had cancer. They just took my word for it. I guess they don't have issues of people faking cancer just to snag the free breast prostheses and mastectomy bras.

God is showing me a side of the world I wasn't so acutely aware of in my pre-cancerous days. There are caring people with sincere empathy and generosity that are surrounding me with wise and gentle counsel and love. Friends, many of whom I see very rarely, are showering me with gifts, and notes, and offers of help. When God tells us we are not alone, He doesn't mean *only He* is with us. He *is* always with us, of course, but so are those He has prepared to be further sources of comfort and compassion. I am not alone. You are not alone.

The other lesson He is driving home: the best thing to do with your own pain is help others in similar situations.

One of the moms I work with told me early on that no one cares about her and she has no one to turn to. I pointed her to God first, but have felt a deep obligation to touch base with her regularly. Nobody wants to feel that no one in the world cares about them. I have been on the receiving end of a flood of love from others. I know how important it is to know God is there, but we are humans and need fellow humans to care about us too! I shouldn't expect it *from* others if I am not willing to be that loving friend *to* others.

I guess that's the Golden Rule. If you want to *see* the blessing of God, *be* a blessing of God.

I came home, and made myself healthy bone-broth soup with lots of yummy vegetables. While sipping my healthy lunch, I glanced at the mirror. *Yikes! That hair is short!* The good news is if I do need chemo, going bald won't be such a shock.

And then, my friend Carol, one of the kindest people on earth who I think has given me a gift every day since my diagnosis, showed up with flowers. I told her she'd be in my blog because she is doing EXACTLY what I am talking about. I think the Bible should have a new verse: *Go ye therefore, and be like Carol.*

I have about a hundred friends and family being the hands and feet of Jesus to me during this rough patch. Thank you, all of you. The prayers, the love, the notes, the support means the world to me.

Romans 11:1-5

I ask, then, has God rejected his people? By no means! For I myself am an Israelite, a descendant of Abraham, a member of the tribe of Benjamin. God has not rejected his people whom he foreknew. Do you not know what the Scripture says of Elijah, how he appeals to God against Israel? "Lord, they have killed your prophets, they have demolished your altars, and I alone am left, and they seek my life."
But what is God's reply to him? "I have kept for myself seven thousand men who have not bowed the knee to Baal." So too at the present time there is a remnant, chosen by grace.

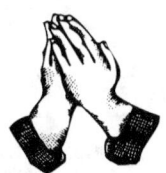

Thoughts on Different Gifts

April 3, 2016

Last night, I watched my sister compete in Australia (on television) in the World Crew Club Dragon Boat competition. They had to qualify and must be *mighty* good to get that far. I was so proud of her and lost a lot of sleep to stay up for the race. Her team was my favorite, but my second favorite was a breast cancer survivor team. They sported my favorite name of any team: Missabitatitti Breast Cancer Survivors Rowing Club. Incidentally, they won a gold medal!

The reporter interviewed one quite heavy woman who was on the gold-medal team. She said growing up she had never been athletic, never won anything, and was never good at much. Then she got cancer.

She started rowing because she was told exercise helped breast cancer survivors. She was hooked, and now, a few years later, she was a gold medalist in a world competition. "Cancer will make your life different," she said, "And you have to learn to live in the new situation, but it is not without joy."

That's probably not an exact quote, but it's close. Talk about someone given a rough road to walk! She was not your typical athlete—quite overweight and dealt a deathly disease. How did she overcome such adversity? With a great outlook that changed her destiny.

One of my good friends and I were chatting about a person with a very different perspective. He finds no pleasure when his impossible expectations are not met in the incredible things he constructs and creates. His work is truly remarkable, and yet he never seems content. My friend struggles to understand why he has to go to such extremes in what he builds, rather than be satisfied with much less expensive, labor intensive, or draining projects.

I have a perfectionist bent, so I understand the personality type. However, I also understand my friend's frustration with him. *Good enough* is never good enough in his world, and those who would settle for less earn his contempt.

Analogies often help me, so I proposed one to my friend. I love red wine, and have a glass with dinner almost each night. However, I am hardly a connoisseur. I drink boxed red wine. I am sure wine drinkers who understand fine wine cringe to read that. I cringe to think anyone would pay $500 or more for a bottle of wine. I wouldn't, even if I *had* the money (which I don't). However, I can't tell the difference between boxed wine, a $10 bottle of wine, or a $100 bottle of wine. Fine wine would be wasted on me.

But for those who know wine, and understand all the nuances of fine wine, there is a world of difference and they CAN taste it. (I would presume...otherwise, they are just plain loco or snobs.) For the person my friend described who creates exquisite beauty from materials very few people would ever bother with, every molecule of his being understands and cherishes each detail of workmanship. He *can't* settle for less. It is as difficult for him to understand those who do settle as it is for others to understand his frustrated perfectionism and intensity.

Tension is created. The wine connoisseur can mock and denigrate me with my boxed wine as plebeian and uncouth. I can roll my eyes at his conspicuous consumption as he washes $50 per sip of fine wine around his palate.

This is why Jesus says,"Where two or more are gathered in my name, there will I be."

He knows that two or more can almost *never* gather and agree about *anything*!

Furthermore, we are all created uniquely, and that is a *good* thing. However, we must be careful. We should not claim our uniqueness as a cover for sin. For example, if I claim I am *better* because I am so much more economical than the connoisseur, or more environmentally aware because my one box replaces his five bottles...then I have crossed over from unique into arrogant.

And if the connoisseur looks down his nose at me, and will have nothing to do with me but belittle and insult because he feels I have no taste and no standards, then he has crossed over from unique to insulting and uncharitable.

This is even more critical in the body of Christ-followers. The Bible is clear that we are all made for a unique and essential function. Nonetheless, we are part of *one* body: the body of Christ. If any part suffers, the whole body suffers. All are needed, and all are created to serve in their unique gifting to further God's kingdom.

My mind keeps ricocheting back to the heavy rower, the breast cancer survivor who never won anything, clutching her gold medal. *That's* how we should be using whatever God hands us. Go for the gold with all the unique qualities He has given you, and be grateful...no matter what.

(For the record, if someone wants to buy me a $500 bottle of red wine, I will not be throwing it out the window unused.)

1 Corinthians 12:12-31

For just as the body is one and has many members, and all the members of the body, though many, are one body, so it is with Christ. For in one Spirit we were all baptized into one body—Jews or Greeks, slaves or free—and all were made to drink of one Spirit. For the body does not consist of one member but of many. If the foot should say, "Because I am not a hand, I do not belong to the body," that would not make it any less a part of the body. And if the ear should say, "Because I am not an eye, I do not belong to the body," that would not make it any less a part of the body. ...

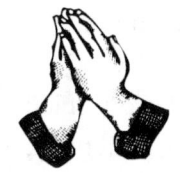

Fading of Creation and God's Eternal Nature

April 4, 2016

My Vinca vine are blooming; a yard filled with beautiful delicate purple flowers. Fitting that our Sunday sermon was 1 Peter 1:22-25. This is about the transient nature of the flower as contrasted with the eternal nature of the Word of God.

The grass withers and the flowers fall, but the word of our God endures forever.

Ultimately, what will we trust in? The things of the world that will all pass away, or God's Promises and His Word which will take us into eternity? If I'm trusting in the Vinca to keep my world beautiful, I will have about three or four weeks. This is a big HINT in which thing you ought to trust in.

My recent cancer diagnosis gives even more meaning to this verse. My body and all the woes of my body will pass away...but God endures, and He promises my soul will always be with Him if I *want* to be with Him. I can choose Him or not, but if I do, He will NEVER let go of me.

In the morning before church, as I do every morning, I sent a Bible verse to the many women I follow who chose life over abortion through our sidewalk ministry. I often hear from them, about how the verse I sent was exactly what they needed to hear. God is remarkable in that way.

Yesterday, the mama I counseled and met only a week ago responded to my text. When I met her, I had promised her I would send her a Bible verse every day, unless something extreme prevented me being able to do so.

Here is her response to my Bible verse text: *Thank you Vicky. You are a woman of your word. I appreciate you sending me the Bible verses everyday.*

This made me smile. I thought about our sermon Sunday, and the eternal, living, abiding nature of God's word.

I texted back: *You're welcome. Actually, I am not a woman of **my** word, but of THE Word. I am so glad you appreciate God's word. So do I.*

This morning, since it is Monday, I head off to the abortion center sidewalks again. I will speak over a sound system, a megaphone, and through cupped hands many, many words to try to convince the women to choose life for their babies. My prayer is the words will not be *my* words, but *God's* Word. Only His Word has the power and conviction and promise that is unshakable, immutable, and transformative.

When I get home, I will sit on my porch and gaze at my Vinca flowers. They will soon be gone.

1 Peter 1: 22-25

Now that you have purified yourselves by obeying the truth so that you have sincere love for each other, love one another deeply, from the heart. For you have been born again, not of perishable seed, but of imperishable, through the living and enduring word of God. For, "All people are like grass, and all their glory is like the flowers of the field; the grass withers and the flowers fall, but the word of the Lord endures forever." And this is the word that was preached to you.

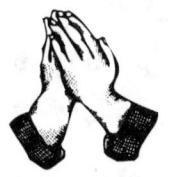

Walking with Integrity Despite Circumstances

April 5, 2016

Charles Spurgeon and I often spend time together in the morning. Here is what he told me today:

Mark then, Christian, Jesus does not suffer so as to exclude your suffering. He bears a cross, not that you may escape it, but that you may endure it. Christ exempts you from sin, but not from sorrow. Remember that, and expect to suffer.

True. I sneezed and rubbed red eyes. Hay fever might not encompass all the suffering about which Spurgeon was warning. However, since my cancer treatment is yet to come, the hay fever is the cause of greater suffering at the moment.

Yesterday was my day at the abortion center sidewalk where I see a lot of suffering as I urge women to choose life. It was an atypical Monday. Few interactions and no babies were saved that we know of. One of the women came towards me, and I was hoping she was going to go on our free mobile ultrasound RV. Nope. She wanted to argue.

"My body, my choice," she said. (Like I haven't heard that one once or twice, or three billion times.)

"Except it's not your body that you're making the choice about. It's the baby's body, which has completely distinct and separate DNA from yours. The baby has *no* choice."

She repeated the mantra.

"Do you believe in God?" I asked.

"Of course!" she said. (Pardon me, but that doesn't seem as obvious as she indicated when about to violently end the life of her own baby.)

"What do you think God would have you do?"

"He wouldn't have me bring a child into the world I can't afford!" (PS- her shining car fancier than mine *by far* made that statement a little disingenuous.)

"Oh really? Where is that in the Bible? I don't recall seeing 'thou shalt not murder unless you are in difficult circumstances.' "

She cut off our discussion then.

Yesterday morning before going to the sidewalk, I read a Bible study by CS Lewis. One of his statements stopped me in my tracks:

God's presence is not the same as the feeling of God's presence and He may be doing most for us when we think He is doing least.

So many of our despairing times or our disastrous decisions occur because we feel God has abandoned us or doesn't care. Maybe He doesn't notice as we willfully disregard what He has clearly commanded. We may not *feel* His presence, but that doesn't mean He isn't there, and it doesn't mean He isn't working. It certainly doesn't mean He is ignorant of our choices to follow Him or not.

As I prepared for my time of ministry, after reading CS Lewis, I read Psalm 41. I could not get over how perfectly God was addressing multiple concerns of mine that would impact me that day. First, look at how the Psalm begins: *Blessed are those who have regard for the weak; the LORD delivers them in times of trouble.*

The "my body, my choice" crowd certainly has no regard for the weak. I pity the abortion-minded mama when she is in times of trouble and calls upon the Lord she claims to know yet so blatantly disregards.

I read on, and came to these verses:

7 All my enemies whisper together against me; they imagine the worst for me, saying,

8 "A vile disease has afflicted him; he will never get up from the place where he lies."

9 Even my close friend, someone I trusted, one who shared my bread, has turned against me.

10 But may you have mercy on me, LORD

Now I considered my own "vile disease" which has afflicted me. (Not hayfever...cancer...but hayfever is vile too.) Cancer has invaded my body, and I suppose it would be easy for onlookers to say I am cursed. My circumstances are certainly not what I would desire but that doesn't change my eternal destiny. Circumstances should never affect our response to God. No matter what, our purpose on earth is to glorify God. We cannot glorify Him by justifying our disobedience to His commands. Or by sugarcoating what we are doing.

Some object to the use of the word "murder" in describing abortion. The life of an innocent human being is being violently ended at the hands of a stronger human being. What else *is* it if not murder? I have been less inclined to sanitize what happens there, especially on days like Monday when there were so many women there to abort that they had to park in the overflow lot.

And now, the best part of the Psalm. The end of Psalm 41 reminds me of why we should rise above our circumstances and walk justly before God:

12 Because of my integrity you uphold me and set me in your presence forever.

13 Praise be to the LORD, the God of Israel, from everlasting to everlasting. Amen and Amen.

If we walk with integrity before God, He upholds us, and we are ushered into His presence for all eternity. How I wish I could have convinced the young mama of this truth.

Integrity is rarely tested when all is going swimmingly. Integrity is doing the right thing when your world is crumbling.

I had packed my kayak in my car, knowing my kayaking days are numbered this season. I have another biopsy Wednesday that will sideline me for another week, and then I presume some sort of surgery after that with 6-8 weeks recovery. Since Monday was the one beautiful day forecast for the week, I hurried off to Lake Wylie after my time on the sidewalk.

As I rolled about on the waves in my beloved kayak (thank you Mom and Dad!), I sang praises to God. I may have cancer, but *I* am the blessed one. I pity that abortion-minded mama who will go home and tonight will lie in the darkness with no one to shield her from her conscience, her actions, and God's presence.

None of us are sinless, but if we have turned to God and believe what Jesus did on our behalf, we no longer are condemned. Sin is overcome, not by our power, but by the atoning death of Jesus our Lord. I pray that young mama who killed her child will come to that understanding. Great suffering awaits her. There are *always* consequences of sin.

My circumstances stink. However, my hope and my goal is to walk with integrity before my God, and magnify His name *despite* my circumstances. Eternity awaits.

Psalm 41

Blessed is the one who considers the poor!
In the day of trouble the Lord delivers him;
2 the Lord protects him and keeps him alive;
he is called blessed in the land;
you do not give him up to the will of his enemies.
3 The Lord sustains him on his sickbed;
in his illness you restore him to full health.
4 As for me, I said, "O Lord, be gracious to me;
heal me, for I have sinned against you!"
5 My enemies say of me in malice,
"When will he die, and his name perish?"
6 And when one comes to see me, he utters empty words,
while his heart gathers iniquity;
when he goes out, he tells it abroad.
7 All who hate me whisper together about me;

they imagine the worst for me.

8 They say, "A deadly thing is poured out on him;
he will not rise again from where he lies."

9 Even my close friend in whom I trusted,
who late my bread, has lifted his heel against me.

10 But you, O Lord, be gracious to me,
and raise me up, that I may repay them!

11 By this I know that you delight in me:
my enemy will not shout in triumph over me.

12 But you have upheld me because of my integrity,
and set me in your presence forever.

13 Blessed be the Lord, the God of Israel,
from everlasting to everlasting!
Amen and Amen.

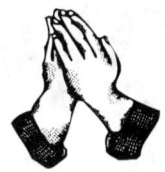

Obstacles and Unclear Paths

April 6, 2016

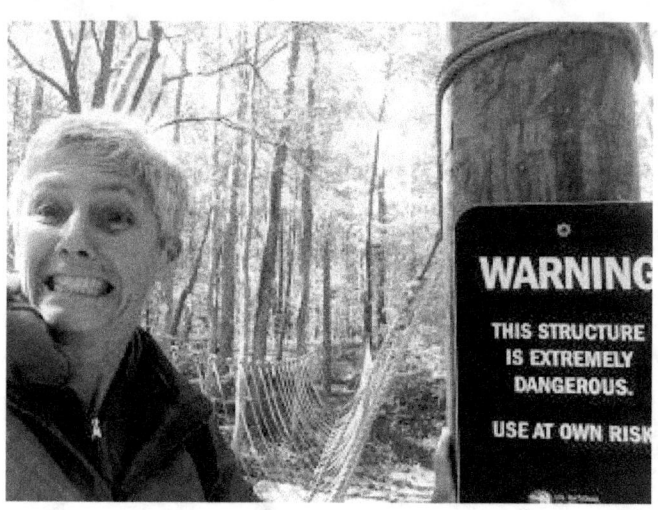

I learned that the practice session for the Olympic kayak/canoe trials was yesterday at the Whitewater Center (WWC). I have wanted to see those for a long time, so joyfully, packed a lunch and headed out immediately. Since my diagnosis with breast cancer, I have given myself permission to do only those things that bring me joy. Life never goes exactly as I hope...and this cancer is a pretty far reach from *exactly as I hoped*. However, *I choose joy*.

When I arrived, it appeared that the Whitewater Center had not gotten the memo about the hordes of Olympiads descending upon it.

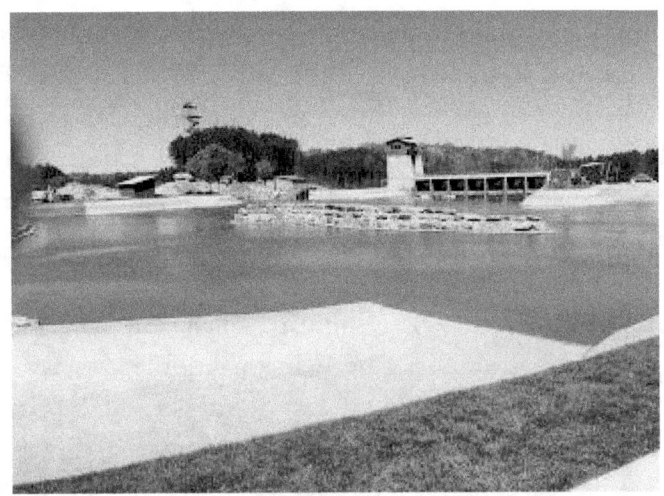

Not a kayaker in sight, Olympiad or otherwise...and the water did not appear to be turned on for the man-made whitewater river. I looked forlornly over the empty (shallow) water. I had already paid my $5 parking fee. Fortunately, I had dressed for hiking, knowing that there were miles of trails at the WWC and I had never walked them! Plan B now kicked into gear.

The trail meanders along my beloved Catawba river, where I kayak. It was completely deserted. I made sure my mace was at the top of my belly pack so I could defend myself against any foe, be it human, copperhead, or Ursa Major.

As you see in the first picture at the top of this entry, there were obstacle courses all along the trail with dire warning signs. I actually took my life in my hands and walked three or four feet on that rope ladder. I sent the photo to my daughter-in-law, who said, "Is the perspective off or is that only about two feet off the ground?"

"No, that is how high it is. But remember, I am almost 60. If I fell, I would likely at least break a little toe." *Go ahead, youngster. Mock your elders. One day, you will be an elder.*

I hiked on, danger notwithstanding.

The tree leaves were newly unfurled, and everything was bright green and teeming with the promise of life. I didn't have a map, and there were many spurs of trails shooting off from the main trail. I could easily get lost...but I did have my packed lunch with me, water, and my phone. Oh, and the mace. I figured with a whole glorious day in front of me and all those supplies, I had little to fear. Besides, there were arrows nailed to trees pointing me along the way to stay on the main trail. I just had no idea how long a hike I was in for.

The views were wonderful and constantly changing. Sometimes I was along the river, sometimes in thick forest, and sometimes in open fields. I prayed out loud since not a soul was around.

"Thank you Lord for this respite and this beauty."

Today, the respite ends. I head in for another biopsy, and then await results of all my tests and my fate. (And yes, the biopsy is *exactly* as much fun as you would imagine.) But for now on the trails of the WWC, I was at peace, and utterly joyful, with clear signs pointing my way.

Ruh-Roh. Clear signs...until they weren't. The next sign had two arrows, unlabeled, pointing in two different directions.

Which way? How like my life this little symbol was. Sometimes you just don't know exactly the right path to walk. Both look equally inviting (or treacherous). I took a guess.

I made the right choice, because I came to a major intersection with trail distances marked for three different loops. I assumed the loops all ended back at the WWC. I chose the middle road, a three mile loop. I know in the real world, three miles is *never* just three miles. Whatever journey you are on, it is always longer and harder than you anticipate.

Fortunately, the route I chose was a beautiful path. Lots of *steep* ups and downs... but it was perfect weather for hiking, and now I sort of had an idea of how long I'd be traveling. I was getting hungry, however, and unfortunately, had to go to the bathroom. Being a seasoned outdoors person, I always pack tissue for just such an emergency and scooted off the path, careful to avoid crouching in poison ivy. (Don't ask me how I have learned to avoid that particular exact situation.)

As I traveled on, God provided a big tree stump. A perfect place to sit and eat my lunch. The river gurgled nearby, down a steep embankment, providing a stunning view. With all needs now satisfied, I put all my trash in my backpack, and started off again.

More danger! This time it was monkey bars with another dire warning sign. *Extremely Dangerous.* I could not for the life of me figure out any way on God's green earth that it qualified as "extremely dangerous"....not even "mildly dangerous". Still, I didn't try it out other than to pose nearby. I already have enough danger in my life with the cancer. No need tempting fate.

NOW a sign for the "Toilet Bowl Loop" appeared. I almost hiked it just to see if there was a real toilet bowl, or if that was the name of some particularly uninviting trail section. However, instead I stuck to the main trail.

The only living creature I saw the entire time other than some birds was a little black and yellow centipede. He was very pretty and scuttling along at a good clip. I didn't know exactly what he was, but I thanked him for gracing me with his presence.

Then I came to a disturbing sign. "End of Loop." The WWC was nowhere in sight...shouldn't a loop end where it began? Isn't that the whole idea of a loop? See. This is what I mean by my observation that no journey is *ever* what you expect and usually longer and harder.

Good news! Although the loop had apparently decided not to be an honest to goodness loop, there *were* still arrows pointing me *somewhere*. I hoped they were guiding me in the right direction. Soon I ended up back by the river, and found my way safely to the WWC.

So what did I learn from God during my peaceful day? First, we all have plans, but God (or something) almost always interrupts them, or downright cancels them! The good news is the new plan is sometimes even better than what we had originally intended.

Next, I learned that dangers exist on any path. Life is filled with danger, and there are always risks. If we avoid all risk, we will miss out on some pretty spectacular moments. Furthermore, the new trails we travel are sometimes poorly marked, or twist and turn, or go so steeply uphill that we are not sure we can keep going. Sometimes the next step is unclear, and we just have to make the best choice we are able. And very importantly: all journeys are longer and harder than we expect, but the rewards are also often greater if we just hang in there till we make it home.

God is in all of it, always watching. If we are trusting Him to guide us, He leads us even when we are unaware of His presence.

Finally, praising Him in the midst of it all has a way of changing one's entire outlook. Disappointment and fear is hard to muster while singing songs of thanksgiving and joy. If our goal is to glorify God, it transforms how we view the obstacles and the path we have to walk when choices are limited.

I sat and rested, having hiked five miles. (I knew how far I'd hiked because I have a great app on my phone called "Map my Run". I was never in any real danger of being lost. I could always follow the pink line on my app and retrace my steps.) A couple strolled by and asked me if I knew if the Olympic kayakers would be practicing today. They too had seen the notice in the paper. We looked at the low water, without a kayaker anywhere on the horizon.

"That's what I thought, too, but it sure doesn't look like they will be here anytime soon," I said. "But I recommend the trails. They are really beautiful."

The couple nodded, and meandered off towards the trailhead while I finished my water and thought *what a blessing life is.*

Ephesians 5:14-20

This is why it is said: "Wake up, sleeper, rise from the dead, and Christ will shine on you."
Be very careful, then, how you live—not as unwise but as wise, making the most of every opportunity, because the days are evil.
Therefore do not be foolish, but understand what the Lord's will is.
Do not get drunk on wine, which leads to debauchery. Instead, be filled with the Spirit,
speaking to one another with psalms, hymns, and songs from the Spirit. Sing and make music from your heart to the Lord,
always giving thanks to God the Father for everything, in the name of our Lord Jesus Christ.

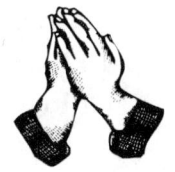

So NOT Fun

April 7, 2016

So just when you think cancer could not be any more fun, they tell you that instead of just *one* lump to be biopsied on your THIRD round of biopsies, you will need *three* lumps biopsied in *five or six* different spots. And to ensure they don't biopsy one they have already biopsied, they first give you a local anesthetic, and stick a wire into your breast that stays in for the next hour as they grope around for other suspicious areas.

Nothing was excruciating. I don't want you feeling sorry for me. But it was uncomfortable, at best. Since the lumps were in two different quadrants, I had to get two different rounds of numbing agent shot into my poor bruised breast. (I had not planned to go grab junk food for lunch afterwards, but as I gazed at the ceiling while deep breathing, and imagining still water and green pastures, I thought I would definitely be getting fast food on the way home. The junkier, the better.)

The doc was actually being kind. If he didn't do that wire bit, complete with a mammogram to determine just where the wire needed to be inserted, I would have had to go on from the ultrasound biopsy to an MRI guided biopsy, with an IV to inject the dye. He told me I was a "special case" and he had been carefully selected and consulted with about my unique issues. Lucky me!

"I hate that I have to do this to you," the kind doctor said, "But I am trying to save you from the MRI biopsy."

"Thank you," I said, trying not to wince, "I do appreciate all you are doing."

"You're being a real trooper," he said, patting my arm.

"Well, I have no other choice," I said, smiling. He really was a nice man and I could tell it pained him to hurt me.

After they did the five biopsy samples, they patched me up, and put ice on me, and sent me to the MRI. If the "tags" they attached to each lump showed they had not made any errors (oh Lord....), I would only need a non-dye-injected quick MRI to check the tags. By now, it was well after lunchtime. While waiting for the MRI, I kept myself amused by drawing pictures on my phone.

Fortunately, when they did the MRI, all was well. Now we wait 3-5 days for results of the biopsies. I said goodbye and told them they were all very nice, but I hoped never to see them again in my life. They didn't take it personally.

I may have gone through all this extra biopsy pain for naught. If all those lumps are malignant, they will not do a lumpectomy. Mastectomy will be the only safe option. But all of them agreed, it was worth it for me to find out and make an informed decision.

For some reason, this thought juxtaposed with my past Monday at the abortion center. No one chose life for their baby through our efforts, which is unusual. Almost always, at least one mama changes her mind about aborting. I wondered as I left, was our being there worth it?

Of course it was. It is *always* worth it to do what God calls us to do. But did God call me to get the extra biopsies? Not exactly, but I was not the one that had held out hope for the lumpectomy...it was my oncologist who said it might still be possible. But I would have to have the extra biopsies to rule out any other malignant lumps. It felt like God opening a window. I could be wrong. Maybe this is just another opportunity to see how much disappointment and pain I can endure.

Or maybe, seeds of salvation were planted in my wake. I spoke to at least ten people while there. I told them all about how I pray to stay calm, recite scripture, and have found pockets of joy even in the midst of all the ickiness, lessons from God I might not otherwise have learned. I chatted with the nurse about my work at the sidewalks of the abortion center, and she was so intrigued she wants to buy my book. I smiled, and joked, and never cried out in pain. God, and prayer sustained me, and I told them that. Maybe that was the real reason I was there, even if the biopsy comes back malignant.

Meanwhile, right before I left for the biopsy, I had gotten a text from one of the mamas I work with. She told me her conscience was bothering her over her lifestyle choices, and she wanted to know what God would have her do. It was a wide open invitation to me to share the Gospel, and God's clear commands regarding the issue she was struggling with. She was so receptive.

"I don't want to feel shame and guilt anymore," she said, "I want to do what God wants me to do."

"That fact is a positive sign," I told her, "It shows you have a heart God can reach. Remember, His mercies are new every morning. Now He can begin to help you."

"We're all done!" said the doctor, as he removed the wire he had stuck into me at the beginning. "I am sorry I had to hurt you, but it was the only way I could help you."

"I understand," I said, "And I'm grateful."

<u>Jeremiah 31:9</u>

With weeping they shall come, and with pleas for mercy I will lead them back, I will make them walk by brooks of water, in a straight path in which they shall not stumble, for I am a father to Israel, and Ephraim is my firstborn.

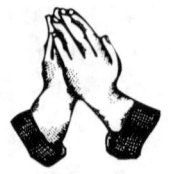

Not Exactly What I'd Prayed For

April 8, 2016

The nurse called, only a day and half later. The biopsy results were back. I prayed as I waited for her to seal my fate.

"They are both like the other ones," she said gently, "Invasive lobular carcinoma."

I thanked her, and got off the phone. Then I told my husband, asking him not to hug me since the breast still hurt from the biopsy. Being a courageous soul, I didn't cry till I hit the bathroom, shutting the door behind me. I guess I was really hoping for the lumpectomy, but apparently it is not to be.

I didn't cry long. No use crying. It is what it is.

My morning reading was Psalm 42:

Why my soul are you downcast?
Why so disturbed within me?
Put your hope in God
For I will yet praise Him,
My savior and my God.

Do I believe these words or not? Is God trustworthy? Is He my savior and my God? Will I praise Him even in this? Yes. I will. I choose God and Hope.

I dried my tears, washed my face, and headed off for my meeting with the radiologist.

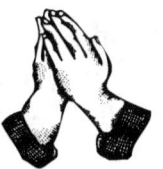

Prescription to Gladden the Heart

April 9, 2016

So, this is my reality: all the new biopsies came back malignant. I haven't yet met with my oncologist, but I am fairly certain lumpectomy is out of the question. The good news is they can now schedule surgery. The other good news is that with a full mastectomy, at least the emotional stress of wondering if every new lump is cancer will be lessened.

However, I did drown in a few sorrowful moments. Only a few. Self-pity doesn't change anything. Now the prayers shift. I need clear lymph nodes and the cancer to not be too widespread to avoid chemo and/or radiation. They won't know that till after the surgery.

I didn't have much time to digest the new information. Soon after the nurse called, it was time for my consult with the radiologist. I liked him even before meeting him because his name was so fun: Dr. Bobo. No one on earth could *not* like someone named Dr. Bobo.

Dr. Bobo was exceptionally nice (as are all the cancer care people I have met.) He asked me all the standard lifestyle questions. I am frankly the last person on earth who should get cancer based on my lifestyle. Thin, eat lots of healthy vegetables and not much meat, don't smoke, very active in daily aerobic exercise, drink lots of water, avoid refined sugar...I told him I *do* drink a glass or two of red wine with dinner, and that the internet seems to indicate this is even GOOD for breast health. If he suggested I should stop doing that however, I would. I awaited his condemnation.

The somber appointment just got fun.

He *agreed!* (Getting drunk is clearly not good...but a glass or two of red wine seems to have health benefits.) Of course, the internet is filled with opposing viewpoints, but most folks say the antioxidants and resveratrol in red wine is healthy, reduces inflammation, and boosts the immune system.

Studies using rats support this conclusion. (My, what a fun study for the rats!) The researchers found that the rats that spent more time drinking red wine not only had healthier hearts and cardiovascular systems, but due to heightened relaxation, refused to engage in the rat-race any longer. (This is just my educated guess of what the results were. You will have to read the research yourself to verify.)

Back to Dr. Bobo and my radiology consult.

We launched into a half hour discussion of fine wine vs. cheap wine. I told him I only buy cheap boxed wine. He told me that the boxed wine doesn't oxidize and that makes it last longer than bottled wine...however....

Recently he traveled to Italy, and went on wine tours. He said he is no connoisseur or expert but he learned Italian wines are head and shoulders above American wines. Upon tasting fine red Italian wines, he concluded they are a whole different breed than any American wine. Italian vintners use less chemicals and additives, letting the wine age naturally. In Dr. Bobo's opinion, that added to their incredible smooth flavor, with no aftertaste or burn.

"Hmmm," I said, "So a fine Italian wine with less chemicals might be healthier for a cancer patient?"

"Maybe," he agreed.

"Could you write me a prescription?" (I wonder if insurance will cover it...)

Interspersed in our wine discussion, he did tell me about what to expect with radiation, and it sounds like radiation would be WAY better than chemo in terms of the misery index. I also learned that if the cancer is not too large, and the lymph nodes are clear, I may not need chemo *or* radiation! So that is my prayer now.

The nurse asked me how I was handling everything.

"Well," I said, "God is still in heaven, and it could always be worse." She nodded.

I left the appointment chuckling over how much time Dr. Bobo had spent with me discussing fine wine. I don't *want* radiation (or chemo...or honestly ANY of this) but if I must have it, I am glad I will be seeing Dr. Bobo. He made me feel like a regular person...not just a cancer patient. And when I am finished with this race I am running, I intend to get a bottle of fine, Italian Merlot to celebrate. After all, the doctor is prescribing it.

From there, I went on to teach my art class of nursing home residents. I had the biggest class yet! I taught them to draw a daffodil, and overheard one of the nurses say, "She's a REAL teacher. Look at how good those pictures are!"

That made me very happy, as did the smiles on all the residents' faces. One of the class members has Alzheimer's. She struggles to speak a coherent sentence but drew a beautiful drawing! Life may not be fair, but there are always pockets of joy. *Always.*

After I cleaned up, and started out the door, I wondered if I had overdone it so soon after the brutal day of biopsies. Weary. Sore. The elevator opened to the maintenance man. He reached out his hand to shake mine.

"I just had to meet you and thank you," he said. "All the residents came down with their art work, and they were all laughing and showing their pictures off to everyone. They were so happy and excited. You did a good thing."

Suddenly, I didn't feel so tired anymore. I cannot change the cancer, but I can change who I am as I go through the cancer. (And if

I can't, God can.) Every one of the residents in that nursing home would prefer not to be there, and most have significant health issues. But *all* of them were smiling as they drew the daffodil.

Philippians 2: 1-4, reminds us that Christ is a comfort, an encouragement, and a source of joy, but that is completed when we look to bless and help others. This is true whether I am in perfect health, or struggling with a terrible disease. The joy of the Lord is my strength, and His love is meant to be flung far and wide to all I come near.

So if there is any encouragement in Christ, any comfort from love, any participation in the Spirit, any affection and sympathy, complete my joy by being of the same mind, having the same love, being in full accord and of one mind. Do nothing from rivalry or conceit, but in humility count others more significant than yourselves. Let each of you look not only to his own interests, but also to the interests of others. Have this mind among yourselves, which is yours in Christ Jesus, Philippians 2:1-4

1 Timothy 5:23

No longer drink only water, but use a little wine for the sake of your stomach and your frequent ailments.

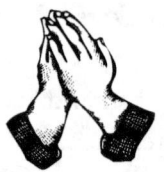

God's Healing Embrace

April 10, 2016

Sheryl, of Truth and Mercy Pro-life Ministries (http://www.truthandmercyprolife.org/) organizes the incredible outpouring of *two years of baby supplies* for the mamas that we counsel at the sidewalks of abortion centers who choose life over abortion. She reminds me often, it is not about the gifts, though most moms we work with desperately need them. It is about the visible evidence of the love of Christ pouring out in lavish abundance.

Saturday, we had a shower for one young mom, "K". I don't want to share specifics of K's life, but she had an enormous burden of struggle and sadness. When she chose not to abort, after meeting us on the sidewalks of the abortion center, her life began to change. It was clear God had a hold of her, and was working a miracle.

After showering her with a living room filled to the brim with gifts, we took her to lunch. She sat and talked about God with Sheryl, Sherry (the ultrasound nurse), and me for six hours over the course of the shower and lunch! YES, *six hours* talking about God. Though raised Catholic, she had dozens of questions about what a relationship with God was all about, who Jesus is, and what He accomplished on the cross. Though she knew the Gospel, she admitted she had never truly understood it...until now.

We had the incredible privilege of praying with her as she asked Jesus to be Lord of her life, and accepted the incomparable gift of eternal life and salvation through Him. We prayed out loud and held hands around the table at Chili's Restaurant, and a new precious soul encountered her Savior.

That never gets old!

I almost didn't go, so weary from the week of emotional and physical stress with all the doctor tests, and visits, and malignant biopsies. I was so glad I chose to go. It isn't every day that you see Heaven flung wide open to usher a grateful soul into the very presence of God.

I left the house at 9:30, and didn't return till 6. There were lots of ways I *could* have spent the entire day Saturday. What a blessing God prompted me to spend it in awe of His spirit beckoning a wounded soul to His healing embrace.

Titus 3:5

He saved us, not because of works done by us in righteousness, but according to his own mercy, by the washing of regeneration and renewal of the Holy Spirit…

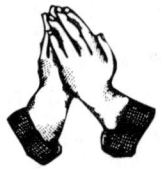

Did God Forget Me?

April 13, 2016

Well, my oncologist called me with the latest *good news*. Based on the recent biopsies, there is now no choice. Mastectomy. Not only were any hopes of a lumpectomy dashed, but he was not done with his cheery new developments. He also said it is pretty likely I will need chemo AND radiation. *Deep sigh*. (FYI- the deep sigh was from *me*, not Dr. White.) Tentative surgery is set for April 20, but it still depends on one other doctor's schedule before they can confirm. (The plastic surgeon will come in at the end of the operation to insert the 'expander' which makes instant bust-line. Well, not *instant*...takes about two or so months.)

Dr. White also said that even if the breast gene test returns positive, he would only do a single mastectomy now, rather than double. He says they must deal with the cancer and worry about healing the known problem first. The second breast may have to go the way of the dodo bird one day if I *do* have the cancer gene, but he says the risk goes up if I whack it off immediately. Because there is always risk of infection or other issues with surgery, he can't take a chance that the non-cancerous breast would cause issues if operated on, decreasing my recovery from the necessary mastectomy.

So, chemo *and* radiation. I guess I will be getting a wig after all. And I was finally getting used to my really short pixie haircut. Now it will all just fall out. However, there is a bright side. I will look twenty years younger in my blond wig. And I will wear the baseball cap wig with the long blond hair to exercise in. No telling what kind of fun that will bring! There are always pockets of joy.

Is it strange that I am looking on the hospital stay with some excitement, happy that someone will be making all my meals, and taking care of me? Sort of like a stay-on-land cruise? I think it's weird. I hope I'm not losing touch with reality...

I called my "nurse navigator" to tell her the latest news and ask about whether someone will tell me how to "look normal" while the reconstruction is going on. The slow expansion of the breast tissue takes a couple of months or so, and thus far, I have no idea how people go about their life without looking lopsided. I am sorry to admit this vanity, but I don't want to look lopsided. I just don't.

The nurse was very kind. She explained that some people stuff tube socks in their camisole...and there are also inserts made for that purpose. She was pretty sure she could snag me some and if I drop by on my way to see my plastic surgeon Thursday, she could give me some and explain their use.

Stop laughing. I know it is NOT rocket science, people, but cut me some slack here. Unless you want to trade places. Anyway, the nurse also offered to show me the tubes that will be hanging out of me for two weeks, and how one deals with that.

"Oh thank you!" I said, "The idea of that part of the whole thing is really scary to me!"

Speaking of scary, there is a really strange line in Genesis 8. The whole earth has just been flooded, and all life has been wiped out. All the humans, all the birds, all the land animals...all washed away. Except Noah and his family and the animals on the ark.

With this in mind, listen to Genesis 8:1--

But God remembered Noah and all the wild animals and the livestock that were with him in the ark, and he sent a wind over the earth, and the waters receded.

Does this strike anyone else as strange? God *remembered* Noah? I mean given that the entire creation on Earth except for Noah and the ark animals were wiped out, did God really *forget* they were still floating about on a worldwide sea?

See, that's how it feels sometimes. Did God forget about *me?*

I did a little word study of the word 'remembered' from Genesis 8. It is the same word used in Psalm 136:23

He remembered us in low estate, and freed us from our enemies. His love endures forever.

That same word, 'remember', is used countless times in the Bible, not in the sense of bringing to mind something that was forgotten, but in showing special focus or attention. God *remembers* His people such as Abraham (Genesis 19:29), Rachel (Genesis 30:22), and Hannah (1 Samuel 1:19). He also "remembered His covenant with Abraham, Isaac, and with Jacob" (Exodus 2:24).

In fact, in Isaiah 49: 14-16, the Bible also says,

But Zion said, "The LORD has forsaken me,
And the Lord has forgotten me."
"Can a woman forget her nursing child
And have no compassion on the son of her womb?
Even these may forget, but I will not forget you.
"Behold, I have inscribed you on the palms of My hands;
Your walls are continually before Me.

God *cannot* forget us! He *will not* forget us! We are inscribed on the palms of His hands! He "remembered" Noah, and the waters receded. The flood retreated. Mountains appeared as the waters drew back, and a whole fresh earth with flood-rich soil dried out, prepared just for him! A new life opened before Noah. God redeemed what had been lost.

Genesis 8:1 is a verse of hope. God remembers us. He has not forgotten you or me.

Psalm 107:25-30

For he commanded and raised the stormy wind, which lifted up the waves of the sea. They mounted up to heaven; they went down to the depths; their courage melted away in their evil plight; they reeled and staggered like drunken men and were at their wits' end. Then they cried to the Lord in their trouble, and he delivered them from their distress. He made the storm be still, and the waves of the sea were hushed. ...

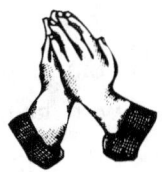

Waiting is not easy

April 14, 2016

I wrote almost 5,000 words yesterday on my new book. I won't tell you what it is about but it is IMPOSSIBLE. Could never happen. It is TOTALLY fabricated inside my brain. And GUESS WHAT? I googled a YouTube video on one facet of my story and it HAS HAPPENED in reality. I was floored. Totally floored. My wild story that was completely concocted in my head has its basis in TRUTH. Knowing this untangled a plot problem and the floodgates of writing sprung open. It should be an easy book to bring to its conclusion now.

Other issues in my life are still unfinished. The surgery for my mastectomy will not be the 20th, as we had hoped. (It is not that I WANT a mastectomy, but if I must have it, I want it over and done with.) It will be later...though I don't know when yet. It gets harder to keep smiling but I am trying.

In the midst of that disappointment, I got a package from my goofy sister, Amy. It is a hat with hair, modeled from the Disney movie *Frozen*. I didn't see that movie but the hat and long braids are fun. It is a child's hat...and fits me great. I have a tiny head. It made me laugh. Thanks Amy. Laughter is important right now.

I wasn't laughing when I called the nurse to ask about my surgery schedule. They had told me they would schedule it Monday...so my hopes were raised. It STILL isn't scheduled, and may not be till May. I know I have an invasive cancer throughout my breast, and I know waiting is not good. I played the "I'm dying" card...but since all their patients can play that, it didn't have as big an effect as it might have. All I can do is wait.

There are lots of Bible verses about how to wait. If I need any guidance on my attitude during waiting, it is there for the picking. Here is a sample:

"So you, by the help of your God, return, hold fast to love and justice, and wait continually for your God." Hosea 12:6

But they who wait for the Lord shall renew their strength; they shall mount up with wings like eagles; they shall run and not be weary; they shall walk and not faint. Isaiah 40:31

I wait for the Lord, my soul waits, and in his word I hope; my soul waits for the Lord more than watchmen for the morning, more than watchmen for the morning. Psalm 130: 5-6

Be still before the Lord and wait patiently for him; fret not yourself over the one who prospers in his way, over the man who carries out evil devices! Psalm 37:7

"And now, O Lord, for what do I wait? My hope is in you. Psalm 39:7

But as for me, I will look to the Lord; I will wait for the God of my salvation; my God will hear me. Micah 7:7

For God alone, O my soul, wait in silence, for my hope is from him. Psalm 62:5

Therefore the Lord waits to be gracious to you, and therefore he exalts himself to show mercy to you. For the Lord is a God of justice; blessed are all those who wait for him. Isaiah 30:18

We are to wait in silence, holding fast to love and justice, patiently, hopefully, expectantly, certain He will hear us, continually, without growing weary, and without fretting.

Is that how you wait?

Me either.

But God, Bless His Holy Name, is giving me yet another opportunity to practice!

Now I'll Be a Tree

April 15, 2016

Before my last appointment with the oncology team (until surgery), I went on a walk on the beautiful Sugar Creek Greenway. I passed a memorial plaque with someone's name on it and an inscription. It was nestled at the foot of a small tree. I loved what it said: *Now I'll be a tree.*

This person understood that as his body decays, it would return to the dust from which it was created. His molecules would nourish the tree planted nearby and in a sense, he truly *would* become a tree.

But, I wonder, what happened to his *soul?* That matters to me, because it matters to God. I hope someone told him in time that being a part of a tree was lovely, but eternal life with Jesus was lovelier.

With these thoughts, I went on to see my plastic surgeon, and my 'nurse navigator'. I have been there so often over the past two months that when I stepped into the elevator, the receptionist at the biopsy center recognized me and called me by name. Just like *Cheers,* where "everybody knows your name."

So, I learned some important things. First, my surgery is scheduled. April 29th at 10 a.m. I will have a single mastectomy. If all goes perfectly, the plastic surgeon will be able to put in the "expander" then and there, and actually fill it half way. That would mean I would wake up from surgery with a somewhat normal looking breast, instead of Flat Stanley. Here is another hopeful thing to pray for. They might be able to preserve the nipple. (I told my friend I was texting at the time, "That's *so* civilized!")

The plastic surgeon said if the oncology surgeon agreed that the tumors were not too close to the nipple, then it could be preserved. I won't know if it was till I wake up from surgery. However, he warned me that sometimes, depending on how the skin shifts as the expander does its magic, the nipple may not end up exactly where I want it.

"What do you mean?" I asked, "Could it end up in my armpit...or on the tip of my nose?"

He laughed and told me probably not that extreme.

Next important object of prayer: chemo is not a *definitive* definite. If the lymph nodes are clear, and if the cancer tumors are not large, I may yet escape chemo and even radiation. Oh how desperately I would love for that scenario to be reality. Please pray, all ye saints.

All in all, I am happy. A friend popped over with a little Noah's ark model. She had had it for months, thinking God wanted her to give it to someone. When she read my blog a few days ago which mentioned Noah's ark, she thought God wanted her to give it to me. I am sooooooo blessed by the most thoughtful, kind, generous friends on Earth.

Get this. As she stopped by and was talking to me, *she* started crying. *I* had to comfort *her*.

"Really," I told her, "I am ok. God is right here with me."

I love you all. I cannot thank you all enough for the prayers, the gifts, the emails, the cards, the food, the offers of help. I am overwhelmed. Overwhelmed by love. God is here. Right here. In all of you. I am blessed.

One thing for sure I have learned on this cancer journey. When someone is suffering, offer whatever it is that God prompts me to offer. It will be magnified and God will be glorified.

<u>Romans 12:15</u>

Rejoice with those who rejoice, weep with those who weep.

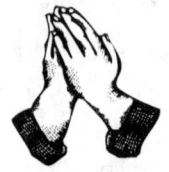

The Temple of the Lord

April 20, 2016

There was another surprise on my foraging through the attic. I found a watercolor with pastel, 22x30, and the title on a little card on the back: *Temple of the Lord.* I don't remember if I used some sort of picture as a model, or if it was completely out of my imagination. Anyway about it, I am somewhat dumbfounded that I did it, and wonder if my talent has dried up. Not sure I could do it now.

Some bad news on the cancer front. Because some of the tumors are right in the center of my breast, there will be no salvaging the nipple in the mastectomy. It was not a huge deal, but seemed to preserve at least some dignity. And the doc is pretty certain I will need chemo. Neither of those things thrill me, but it is what it is. He gave me the same advice I dish out to the mamas I work with who choose life over abortion: *"Don't worry too much about the future, just focus on the next step. Like when I am going into a fifteen hour operation, I can't imagine how difficult it will be if I'm looking over the next 15 hours. It's impossible. I just focus on the next step. Is the area cleaned? Is the patient asleep..."*

The advice was sound and I was *very* glad to hear he makes sure the patient is asleep before cutting into her. That had been one of my unvoiced fears.

Following the doctor's advice, I went kayaking. The *next step* is to stay upbeat and happy before the mastectomy on April 29th.

As I sat cooling off in the water, all alone on the lake, I chatted on my phone with a wonderful mama who I work with that I met months ago at the abortion center sidewalks. Her life is not easy, and she is often on the verge of giving up. But I gave her two pieces of advice. First I reminded her about what the doctor had just told me: *don't look at your whole future. Focus on doing the next right thing.*

Then I shared the advice that I have been learning most clearly since the cancer diagnosis.

Sometimes what feels bad is not really bad, not from an eternal perspective. Nothing we go through is a surprise to God and He uses all of it to refine and shape us for eternity. I have learned that God sometimes removes everything we think we need to show us what truly matters. When we have nothing left to rely on but God, we value God a whole lot more and the thought of eternity is much more compelling and comforting.

A blue heron flew overhead, the sun sparkled on the water, and the river rocked my boat. *It is good, Lord. Thank you.*

1 Corinthians 3:16

Do you not know that you are God's temple and that God's Spirit
dwells in you?

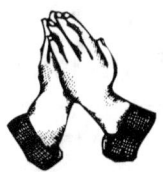

Holistic Approach

April 21, 2016

I have been watching a series, The Truth about Cancer, and gleaning all kinds of holistic advice on fighting this disease. The suggestions I can incorporate instantly that make sense to me, I do. I cannot go into all the science behind it, but there is PROOF that Shitake and Maitake and Reishi mushrooms shrink tumors. I LOVE mushrooms, so right away raced out to buy the first two. (Couldn't find the third).

Next, there is evidence that flaxseed oil, combined and well mixed with cottage cheese, flushes out toxins and reduces tumors. Sounds harmless. I ran out and bought both, mixed them with my mushrooms, and YUM.

I have a week till my surgery. If the tumors I can feel have shrunk, I will ask for another MRI before surgery. If not, I will get surgery, but I will continue to follow the dietary suggestions for preventing recurrence of this disease.

So many friends have offered free products they use to promote health of the immune system. Essential oils, Juice Plus, Plexus. I have accepted all. Why not? I do believe the natural world God gave us is sufficient to heal all our ills. I also believe He empowered doctors to do good works here on Earth, and I trust my oncology surgeon. He is a good man, who called me to see how I was doing, and when I started crying, he told me, "It's ok. I don't mind if you cry."

I do not want cancer, and I am not excited about the surgery or chemo. But I am overwhelmed by the love and kindness of so many people. Cancer has reinvigorated my understanding of how precious friends and family are, and of how selfless and generous people can be in the midst of tragedy. I have never loved being with people. I am an introvert, and gain energy from being alone. But there is a reason why

God tells us NOT to neglect gathering together. I am surrounded by love in my time of greatest need.

Thank you, Lord. Thank you for what I am learning in this trial. Thank you for the unbelievable swell of support by family, friends, and even strangers.

God is guiding us, the path is laid out. When you know the Way, keep your focus on Him. Looking back was what caused Lot's wife to turn to a pillar of salt. Keep your eyes on the Master leading you.

Psalm 32:8

I will instruct you and teach you in the way you should go; I will counsel you with my eye upon you.

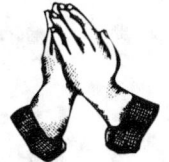

Light Shining in the Darkness

April 23, 2016

Hey! First good news I have gotten since this whole cancer detour on the road to carefree living. I DO NOT have the breast cancer gene! This is especially good news for my daughter and sisters. I think the intense stress over the past two years just did my poor immune system in, and that is why one breast is cancerous. I am vigorously bolstering my immune system. It may not eradicate the cancer on its own, but I am sleeping and feeling better than I have in two years. People, you ARE what you eat. And a restful night sleep matters. (Thank you Carolyn and Doterra Essential Oils: Serenity.)

I was always a healthy eater, but now I am targeting foods known to supercharge the immune system. (Thank you Joy and Alice!) I am consciously spending time each day forgiving the people that I have had anger against, because the bitterness was literally killing me. I have consciously taken every negative thought captive for Jesus because it fuels itself, and despair takes hold far too eagerly. I am making time to do activities that fill me with joy -- kayaking, drawing, biking, walking, writing.

And then one of the woman who I led to the Lord after helping her choose not to abort her child sent me this:

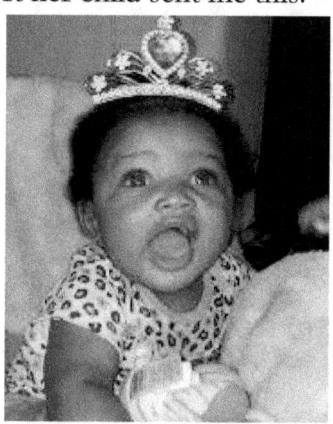

That's a little girl that might not have been here if God hadn't prompted our team to be on the sidewalk of the abortion center that day. *Joy unspeakable!* Also, surely God wouldn't bless me with the desire and the will to speak up for children like this princess only to kill me with a terrible disease...would He? My work here doesn't feel done.

Yesterday, I taught the last art class of delightful girls before my surgery. I told them I hope to be back teaching by the end of May, but it depends on....well...a future I cannot see. We drew a lighthouse and ocean scene. The beam of the lighthouse was the last thing we drew. The focus was first on a somber, menacing sky, then rocks that would crush those voyagers who stumbled upon them unawares. Next, we colored in the tumultuous sea and the crashing waves. Finally, the lighthouse.

Had we neglected to paint in the lighthouse beam, it would have been an ominous picture. Danger lurking from the sky above and the waves and rocks below. But the light changed everything. That beam of light is the hopeful detail that overcomes the darkness.

This was a fitting symbol for my next month. A dangerous rocky shore threatens all who come near, but the lighthouse beam warns and guides. Will it bring us safely to our harbor? As long as we keep our eyes on the light, and heed its warnings.

I lay in the darkness a little while last night, and thought of Jesus, His sacrifice, His love, His promises. *Light of the world, shine on me.*

John 8:12

Again Jesus spoke to them, saying, "I am the light of the world. Whoever follows me will not walk in darkness, but will have the light of life."

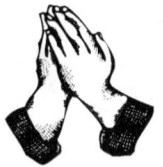

I Am Not Abandoned

April 23, 2016

My friend Alice gave me a whole month worth of JuicePlus three days ago. These capsules of concentrated vegetable extract are supposed to be a super boost to the immune system. On day three now, I can report I feel fantastic. Most dramatically, I feel calm, and energetic. I haven't felt like I was zealous for life in a long time.

It has been a rough two years. I won't go into detail, but cancer is not even the worst thing that has transpired over the past several months.

It really feels like God has abandoned me. It may *feel* that way, but I know it is not the reality. God will never abandon me. Why am I being forced to walk such a terribly difficult path? I may never know.

So for a long time, I lost the desire to live. I went through the motions and I wasn't actively suicidal, but the depression and grief was very deep. Surprisingly, the cancer and real threat of dying woke me up to life.

Friends poured out from every corner offering help, love, and prayers. Every word in the Bible jumped out at me with living tendrils of hope. Every morning I awoke, I praised God for giving me this day.

What a strange enigma.

Now I feel the lumps, with just six days to surgery. Could the JuicePlus and other new changes I have implemented shrink them? Will God work a miracle in time? Maybe. Maybe not. I will trust Him no matter what.

<u>Psalm 28: 7</u>

The Lord is my strength and my shield; in him my heart trusts, and I am helped; my heart exults, and with my song I give thanks to him.

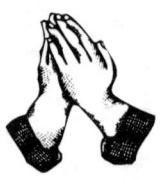

Getting Real

April 27, 2016

It is getting real. The first phase of my cancer journey (waiting) is coming to an end. I went for my pre-op appointment and found myself in a crowded parking garage. I was overwhelmed by how many sick people must be in this hospital based on how hard it was to find a place to park. I had to go up several levels to find parking. Then, I got lost trying to find the main entrance of the hospital. I had to ask several people for directions. I ended up going up or down three different elevators. I wended my way down a convoluted path following signs to the main lobby.

At one point, I ended up in a spooky basement with two doctors engaged in muffled consultation. I mumbled an apology and scurried back into the elevator. Finally, I found the pre-op room. No one in that room looked happy. Including me.

I settled into my seat and began reading the Bible on my phone. I turned to psalm 143 which happened to be perfect. *Oh Lord hear my plea, listen to my cry for mercy.*

The receptionist gave me a form to fill out which made me nervous. Something about listing all the things that are wrong with you or your family makes you think about your mortality. As I checked in, feeling increasingly jittery, the receptionist asked me how much I would be paying today. I hadn't planned to pay *anything*. We are considered self-pay, though we belong to a Christian cost share group, and they would cover everything.

"How much do I *have* to pay?" I asked, worried that I would have to leave them my car as collateral and thumb my way home.

"Whatever you want," she answered. *Really?* That is almost beyond unbelievable. Blessing #1.

"How's $40?"

"Fine."

I paid, grateful they wouldn't require my non-cancerous breast as liquidity to pay for the mastectomy hospital bill. I asked the receptionist if there was an easy way back to the parking garage after I was done with my appointment. I explained how hopelessly lost I had been finding my way there.

Despite a busy room full of people, she smiled and said, "Let me show you." She led me outside and pointed out a much simpler route. I was much heartened, not only by a simpler trek back, but by her simple act of kindness making me feel like I was not just a faceless number on a roster. Blessing #2.

Finally I was called back for my pre-op barrage of tests and questions. To begin, a nurse took my blood pressure. 148/80.

"What! That's really high for me!"

"Would you like me to take it again?"

"Why not?" I quietly tried to think tranquil thoughts while wondering if I would have a stroke then and there from high blood pressure.

She took it a second time. "126/70."

That's more like it! Blessing #3.

So all I'd needed was a do-over! I'd like a do-over on this whole cancer diagnosis while we are at it.

Next on the agenda, the nurse who was responsible for my vital signs weighed me, told me I had an excellent BMI (body mass index) and marched me to the next room. Here, a nurse hooked me up to a bunch of electrodes to do a resting EKG.

"I've never had an EKG before," I said, as she pasted electrodes all over me.

"Really? Well you *are* pretty young."

No, I am not. Still. It was nice of her to lie.

"Nice," said the nurse, reading my EKG results.

Blessing #4.

Now the anesthesiologist came in. I had a passel of questions for him. I am very sensitive to drugs, all drugs. Would I die from the anesthesiology? Probably not. He made notes of my concerns, and explained how careful they would be.

Then he explained the process. "When you arrive, we will give you a sedative. It will be like having a few glasses of wine but without the hangover." (Blessing #5, and #6....maybe even #7.)

"That sounds GREAT," I said, perking up. Maybe this operation was not *all* bad.

After that, I go to sleep. He assured me they monitor me carefully, and can handle any emergency.

The anesthesiologist left, and in came the surgical nurse. She went over all the meds, vitamins, allergies in my life and told me which to stop until after surgery. Then she asked if I had any questions. I DID have one big nagging, haunting question...and felt stupid voicing it. But I must voice it. So I did.

"Will they start cutting off my breast without seeing if the cancer is still there?" *What if God works a miracle and removes the cancer?* Friends, I want you to know I am not counting on this, but I won't discount it either.

No. First they will inject a dye, once I am asleep in lala land, and they will determine the size and extent of the cancer. Then, and only then, do they begin whacking. If God works a miracle, they will scratch their heads, wake me up, and say, "Our bad. You can get dressed and go home."

A world of peace overcame me. Now I can enter surgery without fear. Blessing #8.

On to the lab nurse for my blood work.

"We are going to check your hemoglobin now," said the nurse.

"Ok."

"Do you know what hemoglobin is?"

"My blood."

"What part?"

"My red blood cells."

"Wow!!! Very good! And do you know what we are checking for?"

"Oxygen levels I think."

"You are very smart!!! And who do you think cares about that?"

"The anesthesiologist?"

"Are you in the medical field?" The nurse squinted at me.

I felt like a star. Blessing #9.

As I left, I realized I was no longer afraid. I still would MUCH rather not have cancer, but there are really competent, nice people who seem to really care watching over me. And most importantly, God is watching over me.

This morning, the oncologist who will do all the follow-up care called me. She is very into an "integrative" approach which focuses on lifestyle and nutritional support to reduce cancer recurrence (yay!). I mentioned I had a strong faith, and that was what was sustaining me. She also told me that based on what she could tell thus far from all my tests, it was a "low grade cancer" (OH PRAISE GOD, that is the first I have heard this!) and that chemo was NOT at all a definite.

Pray friends that it is not in the lymph and that the tumors are indeed as small as they think!

As our conversation came to a conclusion, she said, "You said you were a woman of faith?"

"Yes."

"Well, I just want you to know I am praying for you."

Lord, thank you for your gifts! Eternal blessings.

<u>Jeremiah 17:14</u>

Heal me, O Lord, and I shall be healed; save me, and I shall be saved, for you are my praise.

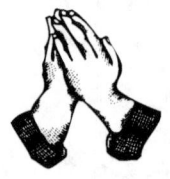

Red Snails in the Sunset

April 28, 2016

Tomorrow is the big day, the day I trust that God has given the doctors wisdom and guidance as they remove my breast, and hopefully eradicate my cancer. I have a lot to do today, including picking up beloved sister Amy from the airport who will spend ten days with me, at my beck and call. I couldn't ask for a better caretaker. She is fun, competent, and kind. If anyone can bring cheer to this less than cheery occasion, it is Amy. I am blessed by passels of friends eager to bring food or whatever I need.

It may be a scary day, but it is day that I am engulfed by the love of God, family, and friends. What a beautiful life I have!

I spent my penultimate day as a two-breasted woman cataloguing more art from my attic, and then kayaking. I was so busy, that I mostly forgot about being worried. God is good. He knew just what I needed and He provided. (I could have done without the 30 mph headwinds on the river, but again, God's plans are immutable.)

Despite hard work battling the wind, kayaking was great. It was, as usual, gorgeous and peaceful. During one rest session, while I sat in the water watching the herons, a skidoo pulled up and the driver asked if I could "watch my boat a sec." I warned him I could watch it drift away, but I was under doc orders not to be hauling heavy skidoos in 30 mph headwinds. He nodded and pulled it safely to shore. (I get the oddest requests...)

I realized I'd been on the water nearly two hours, and I don't think I thought of my impending surgery at all. I contemplated the ferocious head wind instead, and how fast the return trip with a tailwind would be.

Later, while cataloguing my art, I spent more time than I expected laughing. For example, one of the paintings I found in the attic was a childlike red abstract of a snail. Very Matisse-like. Too bad no one will pay me Matisse prices. If I were a *rich* artist, maybe I could pay *someone else* to undergo this mastectomy gig. Anyway, the title is the best part of the painting: *Red Snails in the Sunset.*

Now unless you are of a certain age, you don't get the joke. My father will, because he and I used to sing that song at the top of our lungs on our Sunday car excursions.

> *Red sails in the sunset, way out on the sea*
> *Oh, carry my loved one, home safely to me*
> *She sailed at the dawning, all day I've been blue*
> *Red sails in the sunset, I'm trusting in you*
> *Swift wings we must borrow, make straight for the shore, oh yeah*
> *We'll marry tomorrow and you go sailing no more*
> *Red sails in the sunset, way out on the sea*
> *Oh, carry my loved one, home safely to me*
> *Oh yeah*
> *We'll marry tomorrow and you go sailing no more*
> *And red sails in the sunset, way out on the sea*
> *Oh, carry my loved one, home safely to me*

This song brings back very fond memories, and is a beautiful song. But now, instead of *red sails in the sunset* or even *red snails in the sunset,* I would substitute Jesus...with His crimson sacrifice.

Try it. Read the lyrics and substitute *Jesus* in every place red sails are mentioned.

> *Jesus, way out on the sea*
> *Oh, carry my loved one, home safely to me*
> *She sailed at the dawning, all day I've been blue*
> *Jesus, I'm trusting in you*
> *Swift wings we must borrow, make straight for the shore, oh yeah*
> *We'll marry tomorrow and you go sailing no more*
> *Jesus, way out on the sea*
> *Oh, carry my loved one, home safely to me*
> *Oh yeah*
> *We'll marry tomorrow and you go sailing no more*
> *Jesus, way out on the sea*

Oh, carry my loved one, home safely to me

Jesus is there, the vehicle upon which all my hopes for the future rest. I am trusting that He will bring me safely to shore, despite treacherous seas. All those I love will be brought home safely if Jesus carries them. When we are are safely in our eternal home, we will wander no more. We will have no reason to.

Starting tomorrow, I will be occupied. Prayers most appreciated! Hopefully I will be under the influence of some heavy duty pain killers, and my focus will be on healing. I strongly suspect I will not be blogging for a few days.

Love you all! See you on the other side!

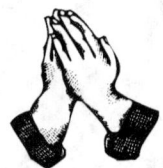

It Was the Breast of Times, the Worst of Times: A tale of two sisters....

April 30, 2016

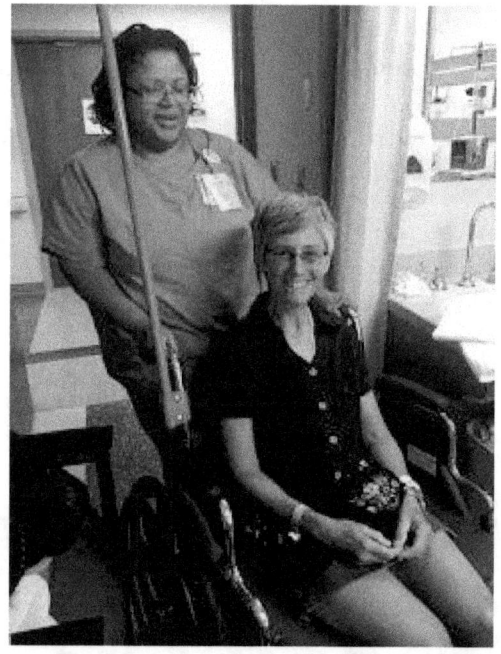

It was the breast of times, it was the worst of times...

That pithy description of my mastectomy was from sister Amy. I told you. She is a hoot.

Here I am in the picture above being wheeled out to the car just one day after surgery. They really move 'em in and cart them out fast for such a major operation. I feel surprisingly ok.

Amy has been a wonderful caretaker. She takes notes when the doctor speaks to me, and takes over the icky duties I don't think I could endure (like regularly draining and measuring the drainage tube.) She nags me ...gently reminds me...about the breathing exercises to prevent pneumonia.

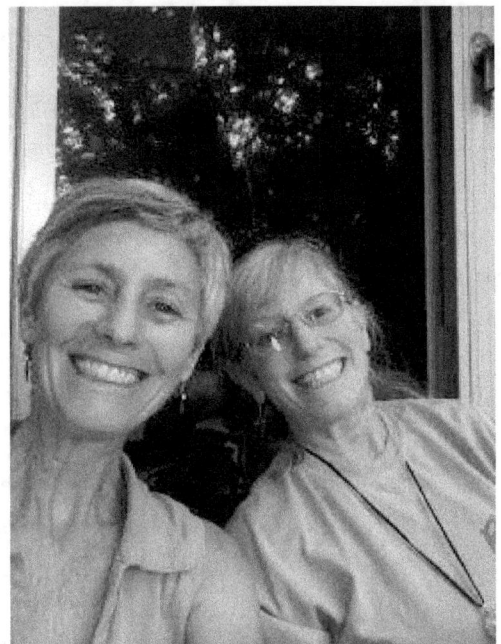

I took one fourth of the dose of painkiller when we got home, and it has been all I needed. The worst part of this whole mastectomy business was probably the anticipation. I had one brief moment of tears when the sympathetic nurse walked in to tell me the surgeon would be in soon. She hugged me, my pity party ended quickly, and from then on, I felt mostly peace. Or oblivion. Both have their place in the surgical procedure.

This was my first surgery, so I had no idea what to expect. I was terrified of the thought of the anesthesia since I have so many allergies. However, they all assured me I would be fine, described with just the right amount of detail what the surgeon would do, and the last thing I remember was the nurse saying, "Here comes the happy gas..."

They had loaded me up with enough narcotics that I didn't feel horrific pain ever. I only have one drainage tube hanging out me and Amy is in charge of emptying and measuring that. The surgeon was very pleased when he saw the output. He said I would only need a couple of days or so on the tube! Yay!

The surgery went perfectly, and they even pumped up the reconstructive "expander" half way, so I look pretty normal in a loose shirt. The nurses were extraordinary, so kind and sympathetic. The nurse with whom I received the longest stretch of care was named Christy. How appropriate!

I have a tendency to see Christ in everything. But even Amy marveled at this fantastic nurse named after our Savior who was cheering me on the whole first night. Amy read the many Facebook posts from friends and family sending me messages of hope and encouragement. Three of the mamas I work with who I had counseled to choose life over abortion wrote and asked how I was doing. Flowers and boxes of goodies from generous cousins were awaiting my return home. Amy artfully arranged a healthy snack on one of the assorted colorful plastic plates cousin Carol sent, "So you can spend time caring for your sister instead of doing dishes."

All the gifts and cards touched me deeply, but one particularly pulled at my heart. It was from a friend of my sister's. She is enduring a terminal illness, and my sister had requested prayer at the time of her friend's diagnosis. I did pray (I often pray for strangers) but I also sent her a piece of my artwork with an encouraging verse on it. This sweet woman, remembering me now in my time of need sent me a gorgeous scarf she had knitted, and a devotional book.

The nurse hugged me before the operation, reminding me that I was no less of the person I'd always been despite losing a breast. "You are not defined by your body parts."

No, I know that. And even more importantly, while I was losing a part of my individual body, a whole host of the Collective Body of Christ were sharing themselves with me. Ultimately, we all drink of One Spirit. The love and generosity we show one to another is the love of the various parts of the body helping the weaker parts.

I may have lost a body part, but the Body of Christ operated in such a way that the feeling of being loved far outweighed the sense of loss.

Thank you for helping me through this, friends.

1 Corinthians 12:12-31

For just as the body is one and has many members, and all the members of the body, though many, are one body, so it is with Christ. For in one Spirit we were all baptized into one body—Jews or Greeks, slaves or free—and all were made to drink of one Spirit. For the body does not consist of one member but of many. If the foot should say, "Because I am not a hand, I do not belong to the body," that would not make it any less a part of the body. And if the ear should say, "Because I am not an eye, I do not belong to the body," that would not make it any less a part of the body. ...

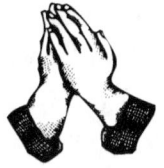

God's Not Through Building my Character

May 2, 2016

My view while convalescing from the mastectomy has largely been looking at my legs stretched out while I am reclining in the sunroom recliner. But since just getting a breast whacked off is not *character building* enough....I developed a very strange, excruciating pain in my calf muscle. The surgeon doesn't *think* it is a blood clot, since I was up and walking soon after surgery... but I can't imagine what it is. After sitting down for a while, when I stand up it really hurts. I can't move. Then I sit, try again, and am able to walk.

Bizarre. It feels like my Achilles tendon is ripping from my calf when I first stand. Wave of pain. Sit, breathe. Walk again and little to no pain. Lovely. Will be calling doc today.

The rest of the mastectomy recovery is not bad at all. The drainage tube is not fun, but there are worse things. Like not being able to walk....

So yesterday (and likely today) I sat reclined, with my computer nearby, and read my Bible, Facebook, G-mail, and napped. It is amazing how much surgery wipes you out. I can tell you that I would be one sorry mess if my hubby and Amy weren't here helping out.

For example, the sink clogged in the kitchen yesterday. I could not have fixed it to save my life. Had I been alone, the gunk-stuffed waters would have overflowed and I would have been powerless to stop them. I would have raised the white flag with the one arm still able to move above shoulder level, and said, "I surrender! Take me now Lord Jesus, before I drown in the putrid flood." And then I would pray.

Perhaps that is God's lesson for this season in my life. I may be able to do very little right now, but I can pray. Now I see why my sisters laughed at me when I said Amy should bring her bathing suit in case we could kayak sometime this post-surgical week. No way will I be kayaking anytime soon. I can barely get off the couch.

But I can pray. There are many times when the waters of sorrow threaten to overflow us. The Bible is filled with verses of God's people calling out in despair as the flood of trials engulf us. Psalm 69:2 says: *I sink in deep mire, where there is no foothold; I have come into deep waters, and the flood sweeps over me.*

In that sorrowful Psalm, the writer can hardly bear another moment. What makes it even sadder is he says he is looking everywhere for God in the midst of this struggle, and his eyes fail. He cannot see God, and he cannot bear life. Hopeless!

Then, in verse 30, there is a shift. As far as we know from the Psalm, nothing changed in the writer's situation. However, his attitude changed. Verse 30 says: *I will praise God's name in song and glorify him with thanksgiving.*

The psalm closes with the writer praising and glorifying God, and claiming the victory he knows will emerge in the end. When all is helpless, and trials flow over us like an uncontrollable flood, praise God. *Totally non-intuitive...*

This morning, the pain in my calf was greatly reduced. I even took a shower, washed and dried my hair, and put on a nice outfit. I studiously avoided looking in the mirror. I cannot yet gaze fully on the poor wrecked breast, though the docs and nurses all claim it is "beautiful." Still, with small glances, I am growing used to it. Praise God for the small daily blessings.

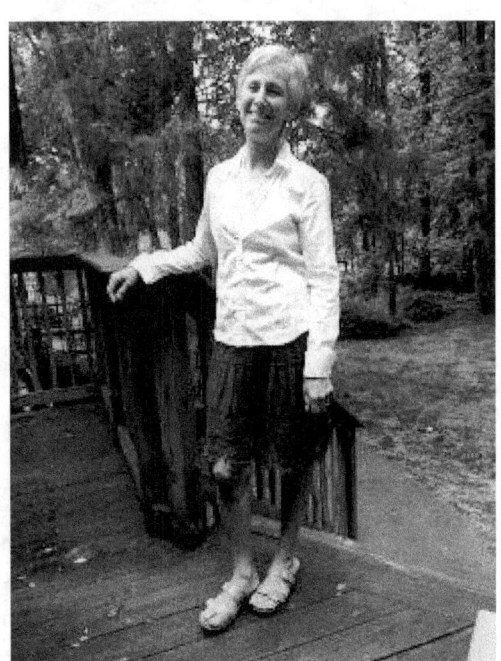

Psalm 69

Save me, O God,
for the waters have come up to my neck.
[2] I sink in the miry depths,
where there is no foothold.
I have come into the deep waters;
the floods engulf me.
[3] I am worn out calling for help;
my throat is parched.
My eyes fail,
looking for my God.
[4] Those who hate me without reason
outnumber the hairs of my head;
many are my enemies without cause,
those who seek to destroy me.
I am forced to restore
what I did not steal.
[5] You, God, know my folly;
my guilt is not hidden from you.
[6] Lord, the LORD Almighty,
may those who hope in you
not be disgraced because of me;
God of Israel,
may those who seek you
not be put to shame because of me.
[7] For I endure scorn for your sake,
and shame covers my face.
[8] I am a foreigner to my own family,
a stranger to my own mother's children;
[9] for zeal for your house consumes me,
and the insults of those who insult you fall on me.
[10] When I weep and fast,
I must endure scorn;
[11] when I put on sackcloth,
people make sport of me.

[12] Those who sit at the gate mock me,
and I am the song of the drunkards.
[13] But I pray to you, LORD,
in the time of your favor;
in your great love, O God,
answer me with your sure salvation.
[14] Rescue me from the mire,
do not let me sink;
deliver me from those who hate me,
from the deep waters.
[15] Do not let the floodwaters engulf me
or the depths swallow me up
or the pit close its mouth over me.
[16] Answer me, LORD, out of the goodness of your love;
in your great mercy turn to me.
[17] Do not hide your face from your servant;
answer me quickly, for I am in trouble.
[18] Come near and rescue me;
deliver me because of my foes.
[19] You know how I am scorned, disgraced and shamed;
all my enemies are before you.
[20] Scorn has broken my heart
and has left me helpless;
I looked for sympathy, but there was none,
for comforters, but I found none.
[21] They put gall in my food
and gave me vinegar for my thirst.
[22] May the table set before them become a snare;
may it become retribution and[b] a trap.
[23] May their eyes be darkened so they cannot see,
and their backs be bent forever.
[24] Pour out your wrath on them;
let your fierce anger overtake them.
[25] May their place be deserted;
let there be no one to dwell in their tents.

²⁶ For they persecute those you wound
and talk about the pain of those you hurt.
²⁷ Charge them with crime upon crime;
do not let them share in your salvation.
²⁸ May they be blotted out of the book of life
and not be listed with the righteous.
²⁹ But as for me, afflicted and in pain—
may your salvation, God, protect me.
³⁰ I will praise God's name in song
and glorify him with thanksgiving.
³¹ This will please the LORD more than an ox,
more than a bull with its horns and hooves.
³² The poor will see and be glad—
you who seek God, may your hearts live!
³³ The LORD hears the needy
and does not despise his captive people.
³⁴ Let heaven and earth praise him,
the seas and all that move in them,
³⁵ for God will save Zion
and rebuild the cities of Judah.
Then people will settle there and possess it;
³⁶   the children of his servants will inherit it,
and those who love his name will dwell there.

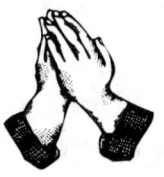

Always Something....

May 3, 2016

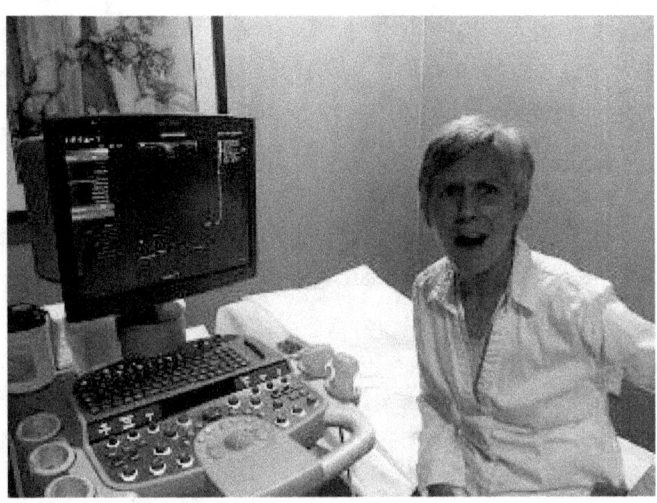

Or, as my sister, Amy told me, "In the words of Rosanne Rosannadanna, if it isn't something...it's something else."

I was recovering nicely, even *spectacularly* from my mastectomy. I was already showering, reaching my head with the affected arm, walking slowly several times a day. However, the sharp and sometimes horrific pain in my calf worried me, so I went to the doctor. She told me we could not rule out blood clots without an ultrasound. She was virtually certain it was not a blood clot. They could get me to a nearby radiologist to do the ultrasound within the hour if I wanted to be cautious and be sure it was not a clot. It was already nearing dinner time by now.

Amy told me I should get the ultrasound. She knew I would worry if I didn't, and worry kills. So off we went to the ultrasound, both certain it was not blood clots, but agreeing it was prudent to be sure.

Guess what? I have *three* superficial clots in my calf. This is better news than deep vein thrombosis (DVT), but still not good news. Amy and I stared at each other, our mouths hanging open. Unfortunately, all my surgeons and doc were gone for the day, and the radiologist didn't want to let me leave till we had a plan. The danger of clots is they can move. If they take up residence in the heart, lungs, or brain, I can kiss my prospects of seeing grandchildren one day goodbye.

Now, superficial clots don't cause quite the same panic as DVT, but the cautions and treatment are the same. Blood thinners and close watching for at least 3-6 months. The radiologist finally reached my doc, who finally reached my surgeon-on-call, and all agreed I needed to bring Amy and take a fun trip to the ER. Amy's ten day visit has thus far included one hospital, one primary care office, one emergency room, and one Radiologist office. She is getting the full pampered visitor tour!

Hubby Arvo, Amy, and I packed an overnight bag, knowing that lately we should be prepared for the worst. As soon as I told the ER triage I was "breathless, and had chest pain and diagnosed clots" they rushed me past the 3-4 hour full waiting room. Now I was honest that all those symptoms could very well be that I had a mastectomy three days ago. They agreed, but they are also symptoms of pulmonary embolism.

I warned everyone who came within 20 meters of my chest that the right breast had just had a most unpleasant week and NO ONE was to touch it. No one did. They did an EKG, O2 levels, and all the vitals, and rushed me to a CAT scan. That was fun. They flooded my IV with iodine, and then the machine takes a bunch of pictures. The iodine causes the patient to feel a sudden hot flash all over the body and then the sensation of peeing all over herself. They assured me I would not, but that it did feel that way. They were right.

Every test came back normal. So the ER doctor told me I needed to fill a prescription for Xarelto blood thinner and see my doc again in a day or two for follow up. Xarelto is the latest/greatest blood thinner. The doc suggested I consider staying overnight so they could do more heart testing. I declined.

"There are risks if you go home," he said.

"There are *always* risks if I go home," I told him.

Honestly, living is risky business. It's dying that would be easy. Fortunately, I know who is and should be in control of that. The Bible is clear -- God gives life to whom He will, and takes it as well. It is not our job to determine when our life begins or ends. Our job is to live each day allotted to us glorifying Him, and drawing others to His kingdom.

The doc gave me a coupon for a free month of Xarelto. When the pharmacist handed it to me, he said, "You just saved $749."

Again, our collective jaws dropped to the floor.

"Next month, and all the months I will be on this *will cost me $749?*"

"Well you will be only once a day, so it drops to $400."

The doc and I will be discussing lower cost alternatives today.

While pondering the incidence of blood clots, Amy and I remembered that right after surgery, the nurse told me I would receive a heparin shot (blood thinner) to prevent clots. She also said I would have compression sleeves on my legs that would work all night, helping squeeze blood out of my lower legs to also prevent clots.

Neither was ever done. They put the sleeves on, but they never connected them. The cord remained sealed in a plastic bag. I had been in and out of consciousness so I wouldn't trust my memory, but Amy was alert and there the whole night. The hospital had not followed the post surgical anti-clotting procedure.

John 5:21

For as the Father raises the dead and gives them life, so also the Son gives life to whom he will.

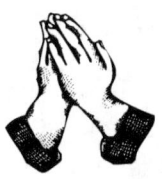

Peace Like a River

May 4, 2016

An uneventful day yesterday! No emergencies or new trips to a medical facility! Sister Amy and I spent the day cataloguing my new batch of art from the attic. This will be the last batch. About 30 pieces. One I didn't remember doing but particularly liked was titled *Peace Like a River*. Bright fall colors speckle mountains on either side of a river.

In the midst of my cancer journey, this one speaks to me. I have not had a whole lot of fun dealing with all the ickiness of a mastectomy and then blood clots, but I have largely felt peace. I don't know why God feels I must walk this path, but if He deems it necessary, I will walk it.

Frankly, I have no choice. What is the alternative?

Speaking of walking, sister Amy and I did two slow walks totaling about three miles yesterday. My calf bothered me very little, so I bet those clots are already being absorbed.

Meanwhile, all kinds of milestones are being slowly achieved. I can lift my arm higher, get in and out of bed without hurling my legs over the side and hoping the momentum will land me on my feet without too much pain, and the drainage seems to be much less today from the yucky drainage tube.

I can even put a loose shirt on over my head. This is no small feat with a 12-inch raw scar stretching from under my arm to my mid-chest. Trust me on this one. This is something I would strongly NOT recommend going through to prove me wrong.

Just so you know, I am not answering most texts, calls, and certainly no visits. Please don't be offended. I am doing really well, but I am not able to handle all the wonderful kind inquiries. My fatigue hits me like a ton of bricks when it hits, and talking for any length of time is very draining. Just know, I appreciate all of you, all your prayers, and kind concern. Bless you all.

As the lovely day came to a close, my doctor called me. I had begged her to find a safer alternative to the blood thinner I was on. Should I begin to bleed, there is no antidote to this blood thinner. As a post-operative patient with two more surgeries in my future, this does NOT bring me peace like a river.

My doctor had conferred with all the docs who did my surgery, and the ultrasound radiologist that found the clots in my leg. Then she did her own research. They agreed that the clots were superficial enough that in many cases, people are not treated at all...just closely monitored. She asked if I would like to take that conservative approach, and do a repeat ultrasound Friday to ensure the clots were not going deeper or moving.

I agreed instantly! This is such wonderful news. The leg is feeling much better, and that was even before the blood thinner was started.

I showered this morning and for the first time since the operation, stood in front of the mirror and forced myself to look. I will not lie. It was *not* an easy sight to gaze upon. I could not look very long. I took a deep breath and remembered breast reconstruction is a six-month process, and each step of the way, I will feel more normal.

I thought about how hard it is to force myself to look in the mirror, to see myself as I really am. I am not alone in this. I think if we are honest, none of us like examining the ugly, maimed, perverted, broken parts of our souls with full disclosure. Yet God demands this of us. He doesn't ask it of us all at once, or we would be destroyed by our own shame and guilt. Our works are "filthy rags" and "the heart is deceitful above all things" and "all have sinned and fall short of the glory of God." The sooner we understand that, the sooner we can confront our ugliness, and be reconstructed in the image of God. But self-examination with the lens of how God views our sin is crucial in restoration of relationship with Him.

I kept the light low as I looked for the first full glance at the aftermath of my mastectomy. Then I got dressed, reaching my arm with the huge scar in its pit a little higher than I'd been able to yesterday.

A little victory. Smiles. Sighs.

This has been a roller coaster past few months, but one thing has remained constant. God has been right beside me, His hand around my shoulder, His peace flowing through me like a river.

1 Corinthians 13:12

For now we see in a mirror dimly, but then face to face. Now I know in part; then I shall know fully, even as I have been fully known.

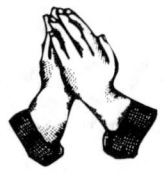

Joy in Cancer

May 6, 2016

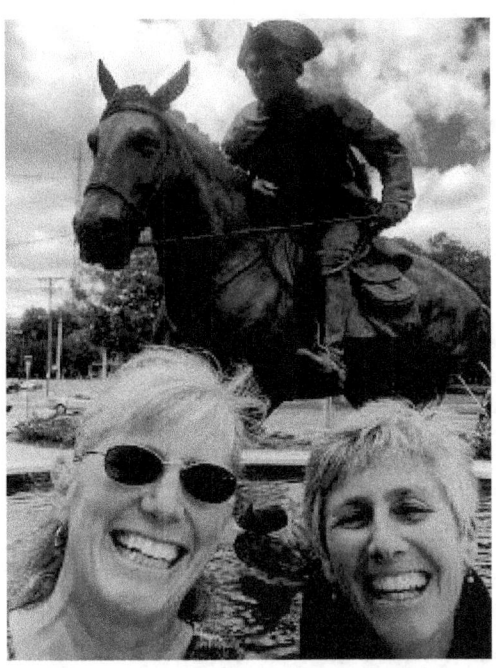

Amy here, guest blogger! This is a test of the guest blogger network. We will return you to your regularly scheduled blogger tomorrow. Had this been a real emergency blog, instructions would have been given. Beeeeeeep.

Long day. Out of the house by 9 a.m. and not home till 4 p.m. , followed by the obligatory evening walk. Visiting sister Vicky is neither for the out-of-shape nor faint of heart. Having logged six miles on the two walks alone, an impressive 18,200 steps show on my wrist pedometer. Darn you, Dr. L, for telling Vicky she could walk as much as she wanted to.

But he also told her good things, so I can forgive him I suppose. He said she is healing well. Things looked good, and she only wanted to hurt him, *'kick him'* I believe the threat was, when he pushed on the location of her three blood clots. She puffed a bit when he touched the still raw incision sites, but it was a mercifully brief exam.

Quite unlike the proctological exam I expect him to give to the nurses and staff at the hospital. Reading his notes and hearing our accounts of what did and did not happen, he verified that the standard pre-op blood thinner shot was not given, the post-op blood thinner shot was not given, and the post-op compression socks were never connected or inflated. All were in his standing orders and all are specifically there to prevent blood clots. She got blood clots. You do the math. Anyhow, despite saying that the tubes would not be out for a few more days, sad news from Vicky's point of view, it was a great report.

We followed the appointment with a walk along the stunning greenway creek path. It winds along beautifully wild landscape, full of geese and other birds, and possibly snakes, we were warned. We did in fact see a snake with a white head swimming along the shore. A Canada goose pair had just entered the water with their four juveniles in a line behind them. We watched in curious absorption as two juveniles ventured close to the snake's location. Sincerely fearing a Jacques Cousteau moment ("and now watch as zee sea monster eats my son, Philippe."), we squinched our eyes closed as the snake coiled in the water and made an aggressive move. Babies and parents scuttled away, flapping and splashing and the snake went on his way too. *Whew.*

We saw metal orb art, statues of heroes we didn't know but still felt the need to pose with, and learned the joy of eating wild mulberries straight from the trees!

Four miles later we were done. The weather was iffy but the Breast Friends charity house, instituted to help cancer patients, was close by, so we wandered there, stopping both literally and metaphorically to smell the flowers. Mmmmmagnolia!

The Pink House is as lovely as the people who staff her, and Vicky scored some needed clothing items. We left there to head to lunch, and here's where you readers in and from the Binghamton area shall understand our joy. We went to a restaurant that serves Speidies! Frabulous day, callilou, callilay!

More errands, home by 4:00, and a top-off walk to be sure that Vicky has sufficiently abused my good humor. Two miles later, a glass of wine.

I'm looking for a clever way to tie in the biblical message, as Vicky always does. My takeaway from our busy day is this: Do whatever you do in the company of those who bring you joy. We never stopped talking, laughing, making irreverent jokes, and praying every hour for one on our prayer list who is in deep need right now. We made sure we followed our prayer promise, by setting an hourly alarm to pray. Joy, I suppose, is the message. I wish you all the joy I have been having!

Proverbs 17:22
A joyful heart is good medicine, but a crushed spirit dries up the bones.

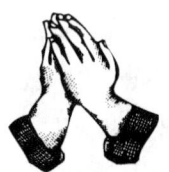

Feeling Sorta Normal

May 7, 2016

I put the inserts Amy and I had searched all over Charlotte for into my new mastectomy bra. Carefully, I closed the bra over my poor aching chest, and stepped back to view myself in the mirror. I looked normal!

If it weren't for the drainage tube, no one would know I had ever had surgery. I gazed happily at myself in the mirror. I have been sneaking longer and longer views of the mangled breast, and slowly adjusting, but it is not a pretty sight. It still makes me feel a little nauseous to see the thick, angry purple scar, the lumpy small swelling of the half-filled breast.

Now, in my new lovely lacey bra, I turned to examine every angle. It looked fantastic.

Finally…Good News.

So yesterday was a good day, the first really good day in eons, with just one minor issue. First, beloved son Matt and dear daughter-in-law Karissa came for the weekend. The whole pack of us went on a 4.3 mile walk to help melt my post-mastectomy blood clots.

After our walk, I had to head off to my repeat ultrasound to see what the three blood clots were up to. Were they plotting a fatal trip to my brain or lungs? Had they decided my six-mile walks were too much for them and finally melted away?

The ultrasound tech said the two deepest (and thus most dangerous) clots were gone! Since I am not dead, I assume they are reabsorbed. The most superficial clot is still there, but of much less concern. So, yay.

However, my drainage tube insertion area was bright red/rashy, and bothering me. I called the doc. It was an allergic reaction to the tape. The nurse told me what to do over the phone to change the tape, and sister Amy skillfully and masterfully made me a new itch-free covering of the area. I feel MUCH better.

But the day of good news was not over. My surgeon called with the pathology report from the surgery. There were only the four tumors they had known about. No surprises. All were small. All had clean margins, no cancerous cells in the margins of tissue removed! One lymph node had one very small spot of cancer but so small as to be of very little concern. The other two sentinel lymph nodes were clean! The surgeon said he was pleasantly surprised. The fairly rosy picture is not what he expected. While radiation is still probably called for, he is cautiously optimistic I may not need chemo!

So, after a season of continual struggle and bad news, I could barely believe it. Now, they may still decide I need chemo, but I have the first ember of hope that I won't, and all the other news is very good. I almost don't know how to handle good news. I've come to expect that it will always be as bad as it has been...and I will be given yet another lesson in how to trust God in adversity.

Maybe, *just maybe,* I am being given a lesson in how to rejoice with God in blessings. Honestly, it is an easier lesson, and one I am sooooooo ready to learn.

Philippians 4:4

Rejoice in the Lord always; again I will say, Rejoice.

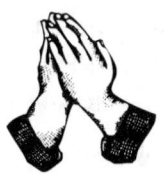

Like Jesus

May 9, 2016

I found a watercolor in my attic stash which represents everything I am not. I am not a great cook nor know my way around a kitchen. It is how I stay thin. Who wants to eat what I make? Usually not *me*. Sister Amy is helping me catalogue and neatly store all my paintings for sale, and was puzzled why I, the anti-kitchen type, would paint a kitchen.

Meanwhile, on the cancer journey there were two developments. I am still logging 33 cc's a day from the drainage tube...and it can't come out till I have 30 cc or less. GRRRRRRRR. Then, I developed yet another rash around the insertion point, this time from paper tape holding the gauze. My skin cannot tolerate ANY tape. I removed the dressing altogether and have a call in to the doc to be sure that is okay.

The second unhappy side effect of my mastectomy: the front of my right leg is popping out ugly veins all of sudden. They never did that before the blood clots, which appeared after surgery. When I elevate my legs, they go away, but I can't spend my life with elevated legs. Calling the *other* doc on this development. I am so full of surprises!

Tuesday I meet with the surgeon again, and I hope to hear the treatment plan from here on out. Prayers would be much appreciated. They gave me the hope of no chemo...but I am afraid to hope too fervently for that. Maybe you all could hope for me.

See, it is all the support and prayers and love I have received from others that has sustained me. I would have been *terrified* through much of the surgery and aftermath, except for sister Amy. She was always calm, competent, and gentle. She always advised correctly, did all the yucky tasks no one in their right mind would want to do (such as empty the drainage tubes), and did it all with a smile. I have had FUN this past ten days. How many people undergoing a mastectomy can say that?

Sister Amy has been my accomplice on wild pony adventures, kayaking, biking, hiking, and college visits with my teens. I don't know what I would do without Amy. She models sacrificial love better than anyone I know. When I look at Amy, I see the character of Jesus.

That same sister is now making me banana-strawberry muffins. She could confidently hang the suzy homemaker painting in her home and no one would laugh at her.

I just wish I didn't have to lose a breast to get her out here for ten days...but God in His wisdom knew who I needed, and sent her. I can probably trust Him on the rest of my life too.

Good news! Doc called and said no matter what, the icky tube comes out Thursday!

John 15:13

Greater love has no one than this, that someone lay down his life for his friends.

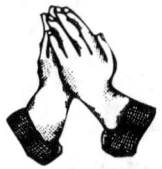

One Last Day of the Angel of Mercy

May 10, 2016

Today is the last day dear sister Amy will be with me in her errand of mercy helping me through the mastectomy. She flies home this afternoon. I survived the mastectomy. I am not sure I can survive Amy leaving.

We went out for Carolina BBQ yesterday at a Southend icon, and enjoyed the funny jalopy on the front lawn. Then Amy spent hours wrapping and cataloguing the last bit of my artwork from the attic. It is now all accounted for, named, wrapped in plastic, and ready for sale.

Today, I see my oncology surgeon, and I think I get the final verdict on chemo or no. Then Amy and I will go enjoy the lovely trails of the Whitewater Center before she flies home. *Super big sigh.* I will have to endure the aftermath of the mastectomy all by my lonesome after she leaves, but she has certainly left me in good shape.

We got the mastectomy hospital bill. $90,000. And that doesn't include the surgeon's fees.

But, here is what astounds me. Only two months ago, I was just like you. Leading a normal life. No cancer. Two breasts. No devastating life altering diagnosis. And then BAM! The worst nightmare became my life. But I never lost hope, or optimism, or faith. God was here and I knew it. *How is that possible?*

I don't know. It is supernatural. It is not possible, yet it is what happened. If you don't know God, I urge you to reconsider. There is a "peace that surpasses understanding" and it can be yours in Christ Jesus. I promise. I know. I have lived it.

<u>Philippians 4:7</u>

And the peace of God, which surpasses all understanding, will guard your hearts and your minds in Christ Jesus.

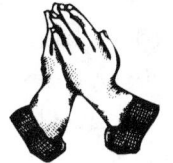

More Good News

May 11, 2016

I had my appointment with my oncologist surgeon yesterday. There was lots of good news. First of all, I would need no further surgery from him. He fully expected after what the MRI showed to find my breast riddled with tumors, and he feared he would have to go back in and remove a whole bunch more lymph nodes. He was pleasantly surprised to see there were only the four small spots he had biopsied and the lymph involvement was very slight. He consulted with the radiologist and they felt I do need radiation, but the decision about chemotherapy will be left up to the oncologist. However, my surgeon seemed to indicate chemo was probably not going to be necessary.

He said I have *great* hormone receptors, which I don't quite understand, but it means that my body will respond exceedingly well to a great medicine they can give me that is highly effective at killing any potential lingering cancer. I would stay on that for five to ten years. It has very few side effects, and he felt very confident that between that and radiation, things look pretty good for me. He said I was healing beautifully and in fact canceled the appointment to see him again in a couple of weeks saying I could wait to see him in six months.

Armed with all this good news, Amy and I walked along the nearby wonderful Greenway to a local Italian restaurant for lunch. We had one of the best lunches I have had in a long time. Then we took a long, long walk along the Greenway all the way to the end. I admit we were both pretty hot and tired when we finally made it back to the medical center, but a cup of Caribou iced coffee and air-conditioning healed all our woes.

Finally, the sad moment came when I had to return Amy to the airport and send her on her way back home. I could not have done this without Amy. Certainly, without her it was unlikely that the past ten days which should've been the worst of my life, were instead a victory, even a *joy,* filled with trusting in God and being ever grateful for what He has given me, particularly in the sibling department.

If indeed I do not need chemo, the worst of this ordeal is over. I still have a long road, but I've learned that I can do almost anything when I'm surrounded by prayer, family, and the love of God. I believe that there *was* a breast riddled with cancer, just like the MRI showed, and just like the surgeon feared. However, I believe the prayers of hundreds of my friends and family produced a miracle. Thank you all. I am blessed.

Philippians 4:6

Do not be anxious about anything, but in everything by prayer and supplication with thanksgiving let your requests be made known to God.

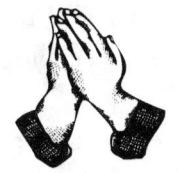

Be My Shepherd And Carry Me Forever

May 12, 2016

I went on three different walks yesterday, for a total of ten miles. I could get used to recuperating. Resting, and walking with little other obligations is a pleasant life, except for that bit about the mastectomy to bring it all about. I don't recommend sacrificing a breast for the privilege, but I enjoyed the restful convalescence.

Just one quick visit to my GP doctor yesterday to check the status of the remaining blood clot. My doctor thinks we can just "wait and see" now since the pain is nearly gone, and neither of us can feel anything in my calf. Otherwise, I spent the day resting, and walking. Walking is critical both to help dissolve the blood clot, and to promote healing of the mastectomy and regaining strength.

The last time I was at my GP doctor's office was two days after the mastectomy, in terrible pain from the unknown blood clots. My blood pressure and pulse were sky-high, and I think I looked pretty terrible. I sure *felt* terrible. This time, eleven days from surgery, I bounded into the exam room, newly showered, in a cute skirt, and feeling downright perky.

"Oh my!" said the very sweet nurse, "You look great!"

"I feel great," I told her.

"Last time, I felt so bad for you. I thought about you all day...just having had surgery, and then those blood clots...I thought, 'This is real...' "

I was so touched that she had felt sad for me, thought about me, and been sorrowful about the burden I had to bear. The doctor was similarly kind. She told me she wanted me back for the follow-up visit, "to lay eyes on you, and be sure you were okay." She hugged me when I left.

There are people who don't trust the medical profession, who feel they are just in it for the money. This has not been my experience. Maybe I am just blessed with stupendous doctors, but they have all been beyond kind to me. Even the hospital business office man I spoke with yesterday told me the story of his own mom who had breast cancer, and he encouraged me with how well his mom was still doing 36 years later.

I found another forgotten artwork titled: *Be My Shepherd, and Carry Me Forever*. I titled it from a verse from the Bible. It is what Jesus promises His children. He will guide, protect, and care for us for all eternity. While we are here on earth, He calls each of us to be more like Him. That *must* entail whenever possible that we carry one another's burdens as best we can. Through my cancer ordeal, many have helped me carry the burden. I have never felt alone, not only because God is with me, but His people are too.

It makes me want to reach out all the more to those who have no one else. So many people feel all alone, and that should never happen. Jesus would never want us to let a fellow human being suffer without the comfort of others. Isaiah 58:10 says: *If you pour yourself out for the hungry and satisfy the desire of the afflicted, then shall your light rise in the darkness and your gloom be as the noonday.*

When we pour ourselves out for others, our own light is brighter. Look at how the verse closes—when we help others our "gloom is like noonday". *Noonday is the brightest time of the day! This* is the antidote to depression—find someone to help. Feed the hungry. Ease the pain of the afflicted. Your gloom will vanish, obliterated by the blazing light of God.

To all those who have been lights in my darkness, I am grateful. May I go forth and do the same.

Today, I go to the plastic surgeon and get my drainage tube removed! This is a huge step forward into normal-ville. I am just sad my sister Amy couldn't stay here long enough to share that moment with me. She was the only one that dared look at the drainage tube for the first three days after surgery. She earned some massive jewels in her crown.

James 2:14-18

What good is it, my brothers, if someone says he has faith but does not have works? Can that faith save him? If a brother or sister is poorly clothed and lacking in daily food, and one of you says to them, "Go in peace, be warmed and filled," without giving them the things needed for the body, what good is that? So also faith by itself, if it does not have works, is dead. But someone will say, "You have faith and I have works." Show me your faith apart from your works, and I will show you my faith by my works.

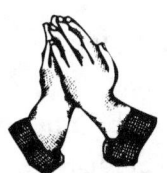

Does God Give Us More than We Can Bear?

May 13, 2016

Five star day yesterday! The drainage tube came out, 50 cc's of fluid were pumped into my expanding fake breast, and I am in almost no pain from the mastectomy two weeks ago. I have been walking 9-10 miles daily, the storm that has been threatening for a week held off for my walks yesterday, and my only job is to rest and recover emotionally and physically. I stopped in at Carolina Breast Friends, hugged the lovely people there, got a free mastectomy bra, and gave them some artwork to give to a woman in need. I felt surrounded by love, joy, and good news yesterday. I am on a wonderful path.

And then, one of the mamas I work with sent me a 3-D ultrasound of her little baby in utero. *What a precious chubby cheeked pumpkin.*

"I am so grateful for everything you all have done," she wrote.

As if one encouraging text was not sufficient, another mama texted me, and asked if I would help her pick out a name for her baby. She was grateful beyond belief that we helped her decide to let her baby live. What a magnificent life I live!

So many women we meet on the sidewalks of the abortion centers tell us their circumstances are unbearable. They know what they are doing is wrong, but they see no way out except abortion. They may know God, but they don't trust Him. In their minds, they have been given more than they can bear, and they seek their own wretched solution. I often agree—not to the abortion, but to the hopelessness of their situations. Most have been brought on by their own poor choices, but not all. *Does* God give us more than we can bear?

Last night, my new oncology nurse called. They are ordering an 'oncotype test' which is a test that evaluates the tumors they removed and specifically determines if the cancer will respond to chemo or not. The results will be low, medium, or high risk for cancer return, and will thus guide the oncologist's decision on chemo. I am praying for low risk, and no chemo. I won't know for two weeks. I told the nurse I wanted to preserve two dates to 'be well' : my daughter's birthday, and a trip to NY to see my sister and folks in July. She said she felt confident we could keep those dates as ones I would 'feel well', whether chemo was in the picture or not. Praise God.

A month ago, the thought of chemo was more than I could bear. I still don't want it...but I know I will be able to bear it. I have borne so much more already than I ever thought possible for one small, timid, pain-adverse lady.

I stopped to chat with a neighborhood friend yesterday. She is a believer and we talked about how often the most precious lessons God has for us occur with the most difficult circumstances.

"He won't give you more than you can bear," she said. As you can see from my writing thus far, I have long pondered this sentiment. It is a partial phrase from a Bible verse. *God will not give you more than you can bear....*

Frankly, I disagree.

I have been given more than I can bear. The cancer is but one in a huge litany of unbearable circumstances over the past two years. As in all scripture, you have to read the whole verse in context. The verse ends noting that God provides the "way out" to endure the unbearable trial. Does this mean He lets us *escape* the trial? That is certainly not what I have experienced. What does the Bible mean by "way out"?

This is where a good Bible Concordance comes in handy. The Greek root of the "way out" (in some translations "escape") is *ekbasis*. (Greek was the language of the original New Testament manuscripts.) This word means *an exit, or an end.* The primitive root from which *ekbasis* is derived is *ek*, which means *origin.*

119

Interesting! The 'escape' from unbearable trials is a word that expresses both origin and end! AND get this: that particular Greek word is used *only ONCE* in the entire Bible.

*No temptation has overtaken you except what is common to mankind. And God is faithful; he will not let you be tempted beyond what you can bear. But when you are tempted, he will also provide a **way out** so that you can endure it. 1 Corinthians 10:13*

Now I am not a Bible scholar. However, I love the Bible, and I read it daily, and when I don't understand something, I scour the original meanings of the earliest most reliable translations as best my meager mind and tools allow.

What...or who...is both the beginning and the end in all of Scripture? The point of origin, and the point where all things end? The Alpha, and the Omega? *God Himself, and only God.*

"I am the Alpha and the Omega, the first and the last, the beginning and the end." Revelation 22:13

This is the answer. We WILL encounter trials beyond what we can bear. I know that because I have! This is the key, and I believe the point of 1 Corinthians 10:13. *God is with me.* If He is with me, I can bear anything because He is helping me shoulder the burden. It is the lesson I am learning, and that is why I can say that this cancer journey has been hard, but not without joy. He has provided a 'way out': God Himself.

Does He give us more than we can bear? Yes. But NEVER more than *He* can bear on our behalf.

1 Corinthians 10:13

No temptation has overtaken you except what is common to mankind. And God is faithful; he will not let you be tempted beyond what you can bear. But when you are tempted, he will also provide a way out so that you can endure it.

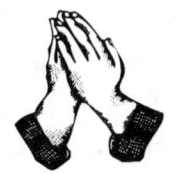

Action Based on Feelings is Foolish

May 14, 2016

While my entire upper right side is still very sore from the mastectomy, I'm feeling so good that I think kayaking is not too distant a possibility. So I called my doctor to ask when I could kayak. He emphatically said *no kayaking*, and he would talk with me at my next Thursday appointment. He said I can walk all I want, but *no* sitting in the river, and *no* kayaking.

I didn't dare to ask him about the horseback riding trip I'm planning for my daughter's birthday in early June. I can neck-rein with my left hand, so I'm hoping he won't object to that.

But as long as he said walk, walk I did. I meandered all over the place logging eleven miles for the day. I didn't have to worry about dinner, because a very kind friend dropped dinner off for me and bought two of my paintings. I have the world's best friends.

As often happens at some point during my day, one of the moms I work with who chose life over abortion texted me.

I asked her if she was getting excited, as her due date draws near.

"Yes, very excited! I look at her ultrasound picture every day."

"She is so cute. I bet you never knew you could love so deeply."

"Thank you, and no ma'am. I would of never thought…"

This is a VERY important text, and brings some critical things for pro-abortion folks to ponder. I met this mom at the abortion clinic sidewalk, while proclaiming life and offering help. The feelings of the women who go there are distorted by the fright and worries of how to deal with an unplanned pregnancy. They *feel* their only option is abortion, and they *feel* trapped in a decision they know is wrong, but expedient. Here is the important take-away: FEELINGS CHANGE. However, once the baby is dead, he is dead. *That* cannot be changed.

This mom, like so many we encounter at the abortion center, was astonished by how radically her feelings changed. She went from contemplating abortion to being overwhelmed by love for her unborn child. This is NOT unusual. I see it all the time!

So much of what we do in life is based on feelings. Just think a moment. How many truly regrettable things have you done, or words have you spoken based on transient *feelings*? Be honest. A *gazillion* if you are anything like me. Then, the feelings change, but often the repercussions rebound on and on like a dagger-laced echo. Yep. Don't pretend you don't know what I am talking about. We have all been there.

And how often do we consider the consequences of our actions/words based on feelings? Even *earthly* consequences...let alone *eternal* consequences. Feelings are not to be trusted. Life-altering decisions should never be based on feelings. Our actions should always be based on conviction and *truth*.

So, where do we find truth?

Fortunately, the Bible is replete with verses about truth and where to find it. Here is my summary gleaned from 62 verses that use the word truth:

Jesus is the Truth, the truth sets us free, truth guides and sanctifies, God is near when we call on Him in truth, His word is truth, we must not love in talk but in deed and truth, we in Christ are in truth and truth is in Him in us, in Christ we can know the spirit of truth, repentance leads to a knowledge of truth, the gospel of salvation is truth, we walk in the truth when we obey God's commands, knowledge of truth is in accordance with Godliness, those who know Jesus are indwelt with the spirit of truth who counsels and guides them, we understand the grace of God in truth, when we exchange truth for lies we dishonor God, if we say we don't sin- truth is not in us, when we listen to God's teaching we walk in truth, and God's law is truth.

How many of us base our actions of this list of what is true? I know the women who abort their children are basing their actions on feelings and lies, not on this list of what is true.

Pilate famously asked Jesus, "What is truth?" He was exasperated because Jesus would not defend Himself against the accusations lodged by those who arrested him. Jesus replied to Pilate's queries by answering that He was born to testify to truth, and those on the side of truth listen to Him. Clearly Pilate was on the wrong side, and Jesus' claim to deity eluded Him completely. You want to know truth? Listen to God.

The Bible is clear. Jesus is Truth. Believe on Him, and you shall know the truth and the truth will set you free. Or you can listen to your feelings which shift like sand beneath a crumbling foundation.

John 18:35-40

[35] "Am I a Jew?" Pilate replied. "Your own people and chief priests handed you over to me. What is it you have done?"

[36] Jesus said, "My kingdom is not of this world. If it were, my servants would fight to prevent my arrest by the Jewish leaders. But now my kingdom is from another place."

[37] "You are a king, then!" said Pilate.

Jesus answered, "You say that I am a king. In fact, the reason I was born and came into the world is to testify to the truth. Everyone on the side of truth listens to me."

[38] "What is truth?" retorted Pilate. With this he went out again to the Jews gathered there and said, "I find no basis for a charge against him. [39] But it is your custom for me to release to you one prisoner at the time of the Passover. Do you want me to release 'the king of the Jews'?"

[40] They shouted back, "No, not him! Give us Barabbas!" Now Barabbas had taken part in an uprising.

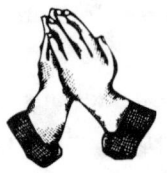

Confronting Pain

May 15, 2016

I am an active person. I can bike for hours, kayak all day, walk miles on end...but when I sat down to do the post-mastectomy "simple" exercises, there was one I could not do AT ALL. The others I could do...barely. What a massive ego deflator.

The Exercise Manual given to me by Carolina Breast Friends was logically organized. The first set of exercises are done lying down, and we work our way up to the standing exercises. So presumably, the lying down ones are the easiest. (Clue to future manual writers: lying down itself is not even all that easy after a mastectomy.) With a little groaning, I managed. Then, I *'simply'* had to put my hands behind my neck, elbows towards the sky, and gently let them wing out towards the floor.

There was **NO** winging out to be had. Not one inch. In fact, I *may* have screamed and alarmed my dog a bit.

I scoured the manual for advice: *If you have difficulty with these exercises, you may need to consult a physical or occupational therapist.*

Well, for fifteen years, I was an Occupational Therapist. So I consulted myself.

"Self, what do you think?"

*"I think you have **zero** chance of doing that exercise in the next millennium."*

"I agree."

"They probably threw that one in there to keep you from being prideful about how well you are otherwise recovering."

"That's exactly my thought. Shall we cross it out with permanent black marker?"

"I sure would, and that is my professional opinion."

Instead of exercising any more, I sat down and read the Bible.

For if anyone thinks he is something, when he is nothing, he deceives himself. Galatians 6:3

The heart is deceitful above all things, and desperately sick; who can understand it? Jeremiah 17:9

Every way of a man is right in his own eyes, but the Lord weighs the heart. Proverbs 21:2

Need I say more? I think the biblical lesson here is painfully clear.

Another little lesson of cancer. After surgery, my entire upper right side was extremely painful to touch. I have avoided church or crowds anywhere because if someone brushes up against my right side, I go through the roof. If someone tried to hug me (which is *likely* in church), I may have to commit a homicide.

Anyway, while reading my exercise manual, it said that the extreme touch sensitivity can be helped by gentle massage with a soft cloth.

Think about this. The problem: Oversensitivity to touch. The Solution: Touch.

Sometimes, because our pain (psychic, emotional, spiritual) is so great, we avoid anything that might make us more aware of the source of that pain. Yet as every good counselor knows, the way to deal with pain is NOT to bury it and avoid it, but to understand its source, and deal with it. Pain must be worked through, till the sensitivity begins to recede. Slowly, even in the worst of pain, most of us find we can eventually find the strength to breathe again.

God is clear about this in the Bible. As long as we sin, we are prisoners to sin. Whatever is hidden, will be disclosed. The best way to deal with the human nature of rebellion and sin against God is to confront it. Opening wide our souls that are trying desperately to shelter our self-image to the healing touch of God is the first step. Admit and understand the depth of the pain of sin -- to ourselves, to others, to God. And then, dare to confront it.

The hardest part of healing my extreme sensitivity was the first few times I forced myself to gently touch the entire right upper arm and chest. Strangely, shortly after I did, the pain began to subside.

There was an additional weirdness of the mastectomy. While the skin around the area was highly sensitive, the entire breast area felt like a numb lump. I have found that the numbness has been receding as I do the gentle massage. I can feel under my arm and my upper arm again, with something approaching normalcy. I can touch my upper chest and gently massage and I don't feel like ripping the sun out of the sky.

The Problem: sin leaves two catastrophic results—unbearable pain, and numbness to the purpose and call of God. The Solution: Admit, repent, and believe on the Lord Jesus. Let His atoning redemption touch every part of you, and be healed.

Who knew a mastectomy would have so many good lessons?

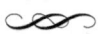

<u>1 John 1:8-10</u>

If we say we have no sin, we deceive ourselves, and the truth is not in us. If we confess our sins, he is faithful and just to forgive us our sins and to cleanse us from all unrighteousness. If we say we have not sinned, we make him a liar, and his word is not in us.

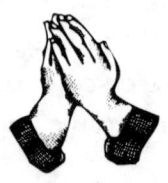

Broken Glasses

May 18, 2016

A large box was delivered by UPS for me. I have never gotten so many gifts as when I was diagnosed with cancer. There was no note or return address to indicate who had sent me the box. Deciding it was probably not a bomb, I opened it.

Six *exquisite* Waterford Crystal wine glasses! Three were smashed to smithereens. What could I do now? There was no name on the box, and no obvious way to find who had sent them, and where they had been made. Fortunately, after tunneling through mounds of packing peanuts, I found the packing slip with the name of the company that sent the glasses and called them. Instantly, they shipped out three more glasses, no questions asked!

Who bought me this incredible gift? I had my suspects. Ever since the radiologist agreed with me that red wine is good in fighting cancer, a few people have been very interested in persuading me to get fine red wine. Thus far, I am still only a cheap boxed red wine kinda gal, and truth be told, I do not own a single wine glass. I use pretty cranberry-red juice glasses for my boxed wine.

Anyway, I knew the glasses came from one of a small list of potential suspects: the radiologist, my sister Amy, or my son and his crafty wife. I was betting on the son and wife. Of all of my family, they are the only ones that could probably have a hope of claiming grace, taste, and class. The radiologist probably owned Waterford crystal himself...but I'd only met him once. I doubt he sent wine glasses to his cancer patients, so that was not a realistic suspect.

Then, upon examining the order slip, I spied my son's email. I don't own *anything* as fine as Waterford crystal glasses, even smashed ones. I felt like crying as I held the beautiful glass. I quickly texted my dear son and daughter-in-law to thank them. They told me if I was going to be drinking fine red wine, I needed glasses that would show off the beauty of the wine.

I'd run a lot of errands yesterday that I'd put off because I didn't feel up to it. Afterwards, I was aching all over. Driving hurts the poor mastectomied breast and arm. I collapsed on the couch, and remembered, "*Oh*. I have Waterford Crystal wine glasses!"

Sometimes, those little pick-me-ups in life are all it takes to turn a wearying day on its hinge. As I sipped my (boxed) wine in my fine Waterford Crystal glass, I thought of Jesus' first miracle. He turned the water into wine. A bridal party had run out of wine, and Jesus decided to help out. In typical festivities back then, the best wine comes out first, and then as the guests get drunk, the equivalent of boxed wine is served since no one is coherent enough to know the difference. But when Jesus transforms the wine, it is the *best* wine. (*Naturally*...made personally by God, how could it *not* be?) The best wine, saved for the end.

I thought about the symbolism of that. Look at what we have to look forward to! A lot of life is really wonderful, but Jesus has *saved the best till last*. *Nothing* we experience now will hold a candle to what awaits us in Heaven "when faith will be sight".

Now don't miss this. If those three beautiful glasses had not been broken, I would not have looked for the deeply hidden packing slip, which told me the source of this lovely gift. The shattered glasses propelled me to find their Maker, knowing only the Creator of the glasses could restore them. How gracious that three arrived intact, so I had a sense of what could be, what perfection looked like.

Are you getting chills over the message God sent me? Folks, we are *all* shattered glasses, created and molded to be exquisitely beautiful. However, the journey we travel invariably breaks us. We have no hope of restoration unless we cry out and return to our Maker. Sometimes we have to work hard at finding Him, but don't stop looking. He is there and He alone can make all things new. He reminds me that when He fills us with the new wine, it will be *the best*.

That's what I thought about, as my recuperating body ached, and I sipped the wine in my beautiful Waterford Crystal wine glass.

John 2:1-11

2 On the third day there was a wedding at Cana in Galilee, and the mother of Jesus was there. [2] Jesus also was invited to the wedding with his disciples. [3] When the wine ran out, the mother of Jesus said to him, "They have no wine." [4] And Jesus said to her, "Woman, what does this have to do with me? My hour has not yet come." [5] His mother said to the servants, "Do whatever he tells you."

[6] Now there were six stone water jars there for the Jewish rites of purification, each holding twenty or thirty gallons.[a] [7] Jesus said to the servants, "Fill the jars with water." And they filled them up to the brim. [8] And he said to them, "Now draw some out and take it to the master of the feast." So they took it. [9] When the master of the feast tasted the water now become wine, and did not know where it came from (though the servants who had drawn the water knew), the master of the feast called the bridegroom [10] and said to him, "Everyone serves the good wine first, and when people have drunk freely, then the poor wine. But you have kept the good wine until now." [11] This, the first of his signs, Jesus did at Cana in Galilee, and manifested his glory. And his disciples believed in him.

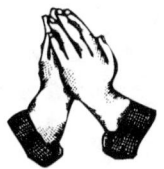

Suggestions BEFORE You Get Cancer

May 19, 2016

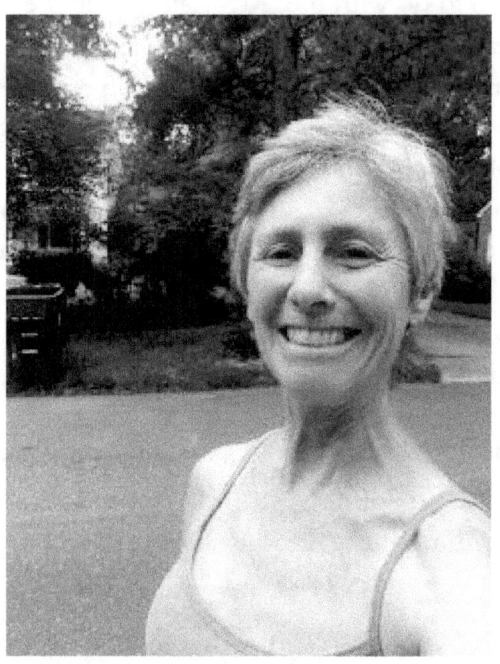

Another day, another surprise. I am going to miss the days of feeling special as I recuperate from the mastectomy. For any of you who are enduring this same journey, or about to: *Take hope.* This is me in the picture above, not yet three-weeks post surgery and I just finished ten miles of walking. The breast reconstruction process is so routine now, and so well-done that no one looking at me would know I had a mastectomy. (At least not as long as I am clothed, which is all anyone reading this will see.)

And here's another perk of breast cancer.

Almost every day, some gift arrives in the mail, or on my doorstep. The day before yesterday, it was six gorgeous Waterford

Crystal wine glasses from my son and his wife. Next, you will never guess what greeted me on my porch when I stepped outside yesterday: FOUR bottles of wine, a horse calendar, high protein flapjack mix, plates and napkins, and La Croix sparkling lime water. Oh, and a lovely serving platter to hold it all. This is from my friend Carol who brings ministering to hurting friends to the level of art. Her ability to cheer others is genius. (By the way, those are fine Italian red wines, like my radiologist prescribed to help me deal with breast cancer.) (Just so he doesn't get in trouble, he didn't exactly *prescribe* fine Italian wine, but he said it wouldn't hurt.)

When I called to thank Carol, she warned me not to drink it all in one sitting. She told me that while she was delivering my wine, she also scared off a political candidate coming up the driveway to chat with me. She did all this without setting off the dog alarm, or waking me from a nap. Like I have told you a million times before, I have the world's best friends.

I would recommend that *before* you get breast cancer, be sure you have great friends and family. That takes time and investment so start building those relationships now. Besides that, be sure you are working on trusting God in the little things, because no matter how good friends and family are, you are going to need to trust God more than you ever thought you could. But you can. If *I* can, *you* can. Best to learn to trust Him *now*, while things are going well. When things go south, you will have a backlog of experience knowing God is always there.

If you are one of those rare individuals who lives a trouble-free life, you can still test God's faithfulness in the midst of trials. Read the Bible. The Bible is a history of wayward, sinful people (like all of us) and God's relentless pursuit and desire that none should perish and remain separated from Him. His redemption of mankind begins in Genesis and continues all the way to Revelation.

I have read the Bible cover to cover over and over again. Long before I got cancer, I knew that the God who created the entire universe had a special love for humans. I knew before I ever had to lean fully upon God that others in much worse circumstances had been upheld by His everlasting love. I was *devastated* to learn of the cancer journey I was going to have to travel, but not *defeated*. I knew God knew before time began what I would endure, and His good purpose would not be thwarted even by cancer.

Today, I was able to shower, dry my hair, and put on all my healing essential oils while looking directly at the result of the mastectomy. With the lights on. With my eyes open. It's really not so terrible.

There are worse things.

Like *not* having family that spends ten days helping you after surgery or sends gifts of beautiful glasses, pajamas, checks, flowers...or *not* having friends who look for the exact perfect gift to bring you cheer along with food, blossoming shrubs, essential healing oils and supplements, or *not* knowing God. He never promised us our bodies would last, but guarantees our *soul* is safe with Him.

John 15:17

These things I command you, so that you will love one another.

Hebrews 4:16

Let us then with confidence draw near to the throne of grace, that we may receive mercy and find grace to help in time of need.

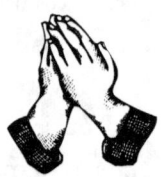

Speak Lord

May 20, 2016

You want to do something really scary? Start adding the bills for battling cancer. One of my books better become a NY Times Bestseller, or some famous movie maker decide he needs to pay me a few million to make a movie based on them.

Or my artwork suddenly becomes the hot new item for the hipster crowd. The disease is bad enough. The *expense* of the disease increases the struggle ten-fold. But it's not *all* bad news. I am recovering well, and the first phase of breast reconstruction is probably done. It is fully "pumped up" now. The next stage is a second operation to even out the lumps and replace the metal 'expander' with the permanent prosthesis, probably in late July. The pain is rapidly diminishing, and the hypersensitivity much lessened. Yes the expander is shifted a little far towards my underarm causing some irritation and pain with every arm swing, but the second operation will fix that issue.

The plastic surgeon is pleased with how I am doing. I was so grateful for his skill in making me a new breast, that I gave him one of my paintings last week. He told me that he was very impressed, and that it reminded him of his own father's art work. In fact, he held it up to his kids and asked what it reminded them of. *Grandpa's art!*

That made me happy. I wonder if he would consider more art in lieu of the the tens of thousands we will owe him? He told me because my skin is 'thin', he thought he ought to do some liposuction to help with the overall final appearance. He checked my stomach and said, "Probably not enough there...maybe from your thighs..."

Now THIS I like. I always wanted streamlined thighs. Finding a medical *necessity* for plastic surgery on my thighs is like Christmas in July. Which is when I get that gift... If I understand correctly, he takes some of the fat from my inner thigh and squeezes it into my reconstructed breast. I don't know why, nor do I care. Sounds like win/win to me.

Probably an *expensive* win/win however...

Back to the good news. I am cleared to kayak. The doctor said pain should be my guide, and he recommends going very slowly and a little at a time. Right now, it has turned cold here, and honestly, I hurt too much to kayak just yet, but I am excited to know I have doctor's approval to do so when ready.

"By the way, I will be horseback riding June 9...is that ok?" I asked him.

He scowled a little and said, "Well, as long as you have already planned it..."

I am taking my daughter and her new hubby to a lovely cabin retreat along the New River, and we are going horseback riding on the New River Trail. I have always wanted to do that, and Asherel shares my love of horses. It will be my last hurrah before cancer treatment begins...whatever it will be. I don't find that out till June 1.

I have been reading 1 Samuel 2-4. These are the chapters where the young Samuel is in the temple with the priest Eli. Samuel is sleeping when he hears his name called. He runs to Eli and asks what Eli needs. But Eli did not call him. This happens two more times, and Eli realizes that it is God Himself calling Samuel. He counsels Samuel to lie down, and when he hears the voice again, to say, "Speak Lord, I'm listening." Samuel does so, and God speaks to Samuel. *Wow.* Unfortunately, much of what God had to say is a prophecy of judgment against God's wayward people. It was not a hip-hip-hooray kind of speech. But Samuel listens, reports God's word exactly as he was told, and the Bible says *"the Lord was with Samuel."*

Speak Lord, I'm listening. Not everything God has to say will be comforting. Some of what He asks of us is very hard. Most of us tend to close our ears to those messages. But if we can trust God with the good, surely we can trust Him with the bad.

I don't quite know how we are going to manage when all the bills are due. However, I didn't know how I would bear a mastectomy either. And I certainly could not envision a fake breast looking so good...and it's not done yet! Each day, God reveals new plans I cannot even imagine, and His mercies are new every morning. My ears are open. *Speak Lord, I'm listening.*

1 Samuel 3: 8-21

Then Eli realized that the LORD was calling the boy. [9] So Eli told Samuel, "Go and lie down, and if he calls you, say, 'Speak, LORD, for your servant is listening.'" So Samuel went and lay down in his place.

[10] The LORD came and stood there, calling as at the other times, "Samuel! Samuel!"

Then Samuel said, "Speak, for your servant is listening."

[11] And the LORD said to Samuel: "See, I am about to do something in Israel that will make the ears of everyone who hears about it tingle. [12] At that time I will carry out against Eli everything I spoke against his family—from beginning to end. [13] For I told him that I would judge his family forever because of the sin he knew about; his sons blasphemed God,[f] and he failed to restrain them. [14] Therefore I swore to the house of Eli, 'The guilt of Eli's house will never be atoned for by sacrifice or offering.'"

[15] Samuel lay down until morning and then opened the doors of the house of the LORD. He was afraid to tell Eli the vision, [16] but Eli called him and said, "Samuel, my son."

Samuel answered, "Here I am."

[17] "What was it he said to you?" Eli asked. "Do not hide it from me. May God deal with you, be it ever so severely, if you hide from me anything he told you." [18] So Samuel told him everything, hiding nothing from him. Then Eli said, "He is the LORD; let him do what is good in his eyes."

[19] The LORD was with Samuel as he grew up, and he let none of Samuel's words fall to the ground. [20] And all Israel from Dan to Beersheba recognized that Samuel was attested as a prophet of the LORD. [21] The LORD continued to appear at Shiloh, and there he revealed himself to Samuel through his word.

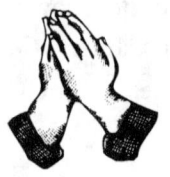

Lessons From Inside the Storm

May 22, 2016

The sun was back!!! After being stuck inside by torrential rain for days, I was able to go on two glorious walks, logging 11 miles for the day. Who would ever have thought three-weeks post mastectomy, after all the fear and despair, worry and angst, I would rejoice in the magnificence of a blue sky, legs that can walk mile after mile, and ears that can hear birds serenading in the trees? It felt great! Up until the sun appeared, it felt like it would never stop raining. Glorious, beautiful sun!

Then, I got this text message on my phone along with an ultrasound picture: *It's a boy!!!*

One of Cities4Life wonderful supporters paid for a formerly abortion-minded mama to get a 3-D ultrasound to determine her baby's gender. The beauty of the 3-D ultrasound is it is so realistic that the mama further bonds and connects with the baby she was thinking of killing. This is critical with mamas who are struggling with desperate circumstances, and are distancing themselves from the reality of the humanity of their baby. The 3-D pictures of this particular baby were blurry, so the wonderful group (Sweet Pea 3-D Imaging) that partners with us agreed to have the mama return and they would get better pictures for her.

Once we know the baby's gender from the lovely 3-D session, we then tailor gifts according to gender for the lavish baby shower we will

136

be providing for her in conjunction with Truth and Mercy Pro-life Ministries. If you are keeping count, so far in helping this one abortion-minded mama, we have three groups working with us to bring her to a place of cherishing the life within her: Cities4Life and its supporters, Truth and Mercy Pro-life Ministries, and Sweet Pea 3-D Imaging.

The chain of loving Christians interceding for this mama and her precious baby was not yet at an end.

This mama accepted Jesus as we prayed with her last week when she agreed to go on our Pro-life RV instead of in the abortion clinic. Cities4Life connected her with a church in her area by the end of the day. The pastor immediately sent some of his congregation over to meet her, bringing her clothes and food. She goes to church with them today. She is excited, and so grateful that we were there to encourage her to save her baby, accept the Lord, and now walk with her as she seeks to follow Christ on this journey.

That is now *four* groups tag-teaming to bring a single desperate mama to a point of joy and hope. Actually, *five*. We first met the mama on the sidewalks of the abortion center, and ushered her onto the Monroe HELP Crisis Pregnancy Center RV parked on the curb, where a trained nurse provided a free ultrasound and first showed her the tiny baby's beating heart. That RV is critical in the fight to stop the abortion-minded mamas. That is where this transformation all began.

This is the way it is supposed to work! When the church body rises up and embraces others, speaking truth and providing for their physical and spiritual needs through a network of believers, God is glorified, and lives are saved. Since I am in a pretty daunting battle of my own with breast cancer, it is a huge relief to be able to pass this precious mama over to others ready to minister and take over from here. One person can only do so much. All of us working together can change the world.

There is nothing like receiving a text like the one I got yesterday: *Thanks so much for everything. Tomorrow I will go to church. I'm so happy. I appreciate everything you did for me and my baby.*

By nighttime, the rain was back. It poured out of the sky in a flood, with thunder, and solid sheets of rain. It never feels like the sun could possibly ever return when you are in the midst of the deluge. *But it always does.* And when it does...it is glorious.

Deuteronomy 31:6

Be strong and courageous. Do not fear or be in dread of them, for it is the Lord your God who goes with you. He will not leave you or forsake you."

Psalm 107:29

He made the storm be still, and the waves of the sea were hushed.

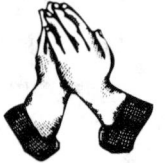

A Broken Pen and a Spiritual Parallel

May 23, 2016

The post-breast-surgery exercises that I could not do AT ALL last week, I can now do. Ignore the fact that I only do five of the 5-7 recommended repetitions. Also, I cannot lie flat and do the killer winging-arm exercise, but I *can* do it with a pillow under my head. If that is cheating, so be it. I am doing my best.

Part of the issue is not the surgical soreness. The new breast is created by an implant under the pectoral muscle. That poor muscle is already being stretched beyond its intended purpose. To do the exercises, it has to be stretched even more. It doesn't exactly *hurt*...well...actually, it *does* hurt. *Exactly.*

But it is not a terrible pain. It is more discomfort, like poking at my eye with a stick. Well no. Not that bad. Let's just say I cannot WAIT to finish the repetitions. My arm is not *very* sore afterwards, which must be a good sign.

Meanwhile, my Surface Tablet Pen broke, right when I have three potential new book illustration jobs. It still works, sort of, so I played around with it yesterday. I created a pretty picture of a lioness even with my broken pen. It is amazing what we can do, even when we are broken.

That was part of our message yesterday in church. We are starting a study of the book of Proverbs. The pastor noted that despite all Solomon's wisdom and greatness, he was as fallible, broken, and struggling with sin as we all are. Nonetheless, he accomplished great things for God. The last thing any of us need to be is perfect to be useful to God. There would definitely be a shortage of people God could use if that was the case.

C.S. Lewis states it beautifully, speaking of God and His work to make us what we should become: *The job will not be completed in this life: but He means to get us as far as possible before death.*

I am a perfectionist, so this lesson is one I struggle with. I need perfection now. (*No-duh!* That aside is what I am sure my husband is muttering if he is reading this.) Cancer is just one more part of the broken world that is teaching me this very lesson. There are things I absolutely cannot do yet with my right arm. I cannot pump out shampoo with my affected arm, or reach the shower head to turn it so the water doesn't slam right into my eyes. It doesn't matter how much I *want* to, I can't. I cannot lie flat on the ground and do the winging-arm exercise without a pillow under my head. At all. Not even close. This lack of skill and imperfections are terribly frustrating to me. The spirit is willing, but the body is weak.

But I am still useful. I can still type to write this blog. I can still go on long walks and encourage little girls selling koolaid (and yes, I *did* do that...), and I can still pray. I can still go to the sidewalks of the abortion center today, and call out to the women, "Please. Come talk with us. Tell us your situation. We want to help."

So I will.

Psalm 51:17

The sacrifices of God are a broken spirit; a broken and contrite heart, O God, you will not despise.

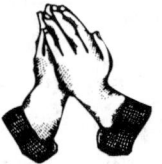

More Hard Decisions

May 24, 2016

So, breast lift surgery on normal breast or not?

I don't like the idea at all of cutting into living, healthy tissue. However, I do look ridiculous without a bra. One breast, the new one, still in process, is perky and taut, and high. The normal breast is droopy and flops about four inches lower and flatter than the new one.

Not many people will ever see me without clothes and a bra...just me and my mirror. Is it worth the pain and suffering and potential complications?

On the other hand, I will already be doing what is the riskiest part of it all – the anesthesia and surgery to the right breast. Sometime in July, the expander must be removed, the silicone implant placed, and the lumpiness of the new breast evened out. I think Dr. L said he will use fat from my thighs for that process, but I need to pin him down on that.

I have a chance to look "normal." Is it worth the cost? I will commence praying and see if God reveals an obvious answer.

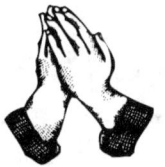

Writing My Own Ending

May 25, 2016

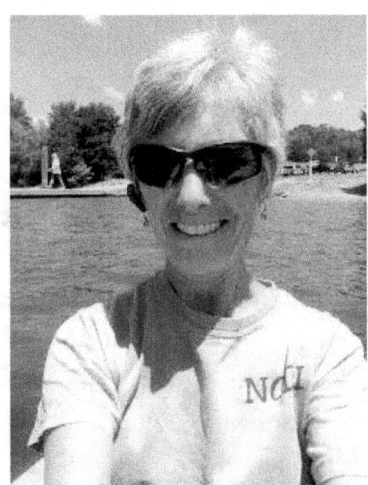

That happy me is 3 1/2 weeks post-mastectomy out in my kayak for the first time since surgery. I went really slowly, and stayed close to the dock, but it felt wonderful. Well, there were sudden sharp twinges if I stroked too hard, but I quickly figured out I had to do shallow, small strokes with the paddle and then all was well.

Still, my shoulders ached after only half an hour, and I knew it was best to ease slowly back into kayaking. The doctor had mentioned it might not be easy since the muscle used in reconstructing the breast was the very muscle used in kayaking. I found the pectoral muscle not so much to be the problem as my shoulder muscles, which must have atrophied in the four weeks since I last used them much.

On the way home from kayaking, I passed my favorite greenway, so stopped to go for a short walk in the shady forested path. As I walked, I felt about as happy as I have ever been. Nature, fresh air, sunshine all have a way of chasing even the most troublesome concerns away. Instead of worrying about all the uncertainties of tomorrow, I found myself thanking God for the sun dappled leaves, the shade cast from the beautiful trees, the strength of my body despite all the trauma it has had to endure lately. There is always cause for rejoicing in the Lord.

This recovery is a nice life. I have doctors' orders to exercise, eat really healthy food, and rest, while reducing stress. And I'm not supposed to vacuum for six weeks. Can you think of a better recipe for happiness?

When I got home, I wrote 3,000 more words on my new novel, making myself tear up with what the heroine is about to undergo. Then I heard from one of the mamas I work with who chose life over abortion. Like most of the mamas I counsel, her background is riddled with trauma and despair. Yet she told me she and the baby's father are reconciling, and they are both going to church every weekend! They both eagerly await the baby's imminent birth. She is a talented writer, and I encouraged her again to write a book about her experience. Her transformation from despair to hope could inspire many.

She thanked me for believing in her but said she couldn't write it, "Until I know how it will end."

"It won't end till we are in heaven with Jesus, and then it will be too late. Write it now," I advised, "In fact, write it with the ending you hope for. See how close the real ending comes."

I did that with my first book about our rescue dog, Honeybun. I actually wrote the ending of that true story *before* the ending happened in real life. I wrote what I thought would be the perfect though improbable ending. Guess what? It happened almost *exactly* as I wrote it. I didn't have to revise much of my make-believe ending at all!

Now don't think I am saying that I can change events like God can. What I am saying is that optimism, hope, and planning for a certain outcome can very often bring you closer to the future you envision. God must be in the center of those plans, but if your will aligns with His, and you have a goal, and steer towards that goal, it is much more likely you will hit it than if you have no clear finish line or plan.

Here's a Biblical example. David was a young shepherd when he came upon his brothers and fellow Israelites cowering in the face of the Philistine giant, Goliath. Instantly, David forged a plan based on what he knew of God. He didn't let fear, the counsel of naysayers, youth, or inexperience alter what he was certain should be the course of action. He envisioned the outcome. And then he did it.

It ended just as he hoped. Goliath was defeated, and God was glorified.

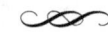

1 Samuel 17: 32-37

And David said to Saul, "Let no man's heart fail because of him. Your servant will go and fight with this Philistine." 33 And Saul said to David, "You are not able to go against this Philistine to fight with him, for you are but a youth, and he has been a man of war from his youth." 34 But David said to Saul, "Your servant used to keep sheep for his father. And when there came a lion, or a bear, and took a lamb from the flock, 35 I went after him and struck him and delivered it out of his mouth. And if he arose against me, I caught him by his beard and struck him and killed him. 36 Your servant has struck down both lions and bears, and this uncircumcised Philistine shall be like one of them, for he has defied the armies of the living God." 37 And David said, "The Lord who delivered me from the paw of the lion and from the paw of the bear will deliver me from the hand of this Philistine." And Saul said to David, "Go, and the Lord be with you.

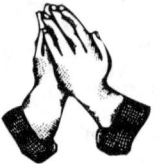

Preparing for Round Two

May 27, 2016

Progress Report on the mastectomy front: as of yesterday, I am all "filled" so that the muscle with the expander is now stretched as far as it has to stretch. Now, the next month is spent letting the muscle realize it must relax, and then I go through a second surgery. In surgery #2, the expander is replaced with a permanent implant, fat from my thighs squished into my breast to make it look nice and smooth, and if I want it, the "normal" breast can get a facelift to match the new one. Not sure if I am willing to shell out $5,000 for that bit of nonessential vanity. The surgery is no cake walk—it is still a three hour ordeal, but I am told not as bad as the mastectomy itself.

My doctor was pleased to learn I had kayaked a couple of days ago. The more I use my arms and muscles, the more I will heal and hopefully, without limitations on range of motion.

However, all was not rosy yesterday. On an advisory note, *always* read your hospital bills line by line. I was charged for two drainage tubes (not cheap) when I only had one, and two breast implants

($5000 each!!!!) when I only had one. They also charged me for the compression stocking to prevent blood clots...which they never used! (You may recall from earlier blogs that there are three anti-clot procedures they do with breast cancer patients undergoing surgery. NONE were done for me, and I did develop blood clots. Praise God I didn't die...but it was still an enormous expense I shouldn't have had.)

Another disturbing addendum yesterday: the pathology report. This was two pages long with incomprehensible names of things that made no sense to me. I read it line by line anyway. On the second page, it noted a total of four biopsies on my neck, scalp and shoulder. This was news to me! I wonder how they accomplished those biopsies with no wounds, and without me knowing. Then, listen to this: based on those biopsies, the report added diagnoses of basal cell carcinoma, and squamous cell carcinoma. This was a month ago, yet if these were *my* biopsies and diagnoses, no one has informed me yet!

Given escalating issues, I called Patient Care Advocates. They assure me they will investigate all my concerns and get back to me.

Fortunately, yesterday was also filled with joyful events. I went on the first run since my surgery. I ran 5 1/2 miles, and then walked another two or so to cool down. It felt great. It didn't hurt at all, except for a few little twinges when I was too vigorous with my arm swings. While I will win no races, my time was not too dismal.

After returning from my final breast "fill-up", I went on the first bike ride since the mastectomy. I only rode for a little under an hour, but it again proved to me I could. It didn't hurt, not even the uphills. I have a lot left to endure, but the milestones each day of cancer survival are monumental.

This is an important key to contentment that cancer is teaching me. The process of recovery and treatment is long, and involves slow progress at times, and long periods of waiting. Since each stage must be healed and completed before the next stage can begin, it cannot be rushed. Every victory, no matter how small must be noticed and celebrated. Things I took for granted, simple things, I now find myself praising God for...and meaning it! Like eyebrows. I dread chemo for many reasons, but losing my eyebrows which I never cared one whit about is very disturbing to me.

This is the way I should have lived all along. What if every day, as soon as I awoke, I listed with gratitude to God all I should be thankful for? Opening my eyes, walking unaided, putting on my clothes myself, seeing the sunshine, seeing the rainfall, hearing the birds, sitting in my own home, reading the Bible, tasting the coffee, smelling the roses...etc.

That list would take every moment to honestly complete. If my heart were so swelled with all the praise I should be lifting up to God, there would not be a single moment for despair or complaining. I hate that it takes enormous loss to gain perspective on what really matters, but so often, it does.

Psalm 95:1-11

Oh come, let us sing to the Lord; let us make a joyful noise to the
rock of our salvation! Let us come into his presence with
thanksgiving; let us make a joyful noise to him with songs of praise!
For the Lord is a great God, and a great King above all gods. In his
hand are the depths of the earth; the heights of the mountains are his
also. The sea is his, for he made it, and his hands formed the dry land.

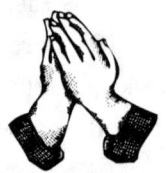

The Peace of God Trampled Upon

May 29, 2016

My husband surprised me yesterday.

"Shall we go kayaking?" he asked.

I blinked. "You mean...*me and you?*"

See, hubby is not really keen on kayaking. I know of very few people who enjoy kayaking as much as I. I don't go for any of the thrills, speed, or even exercise...I kayak because it is peaceful and beautiful. I kayak because I see God's creatures all around me, and I love them. I kayak because the water sings, and rocks, and smells wholesome and pure and good. I kayak because my muscles enjoy the rhythm and movement which they were designed for, and my lungs fill fully with fresh air God has surrounded our unlikely planet with. When I kayak, I feel God's presence.

"Yes, if you want to," hubby said.

So he loaded the car with our two kayaks and we went to Lake Wylie. As I feared on this holiday weekend, it was mobbed. Everyone and his brother was on the lake in gas-guzzling motorboats and jet-skis. I will freely admit my bias. I *hate* motorboats and jet-skis. They pollute the lake, the air, and the sound barrier. If I could ban them, I would. There is a sign at the launch site that fishermen may fish, but are strongly advised not to eat more than one fish a week caught in Lake Wylie due to pollution.

My parents were great parents, and they taught me one thing supremely well. The world is full of free, non-polluting activities that feed the body and soul. Do *them*. So they taught me to sail, bike ride, skate, canoe, run, play tennis, cross-country ski, and enjoy long walks. All free. None use any fossil fuel or pollute the environment.

I tried desperately to teach my children that same value. I don't know if I succeeded. One for sure begged me over and over to rent a jet-ski. I refused. Firstly, I couldn't afford it. Secondly, I am morally opposed.

That's a strong position I am taking, isn't it?

But do you know what happens on holiday weekends when the jet-skis and motor boats are churning the waters, fouling the air with diesel fuel, and overpowering the sounds of the birds? The wildlife vanishes. The fresh smell of the water or hamburgers being grilled on the shore is drenched instead with the smell of exhaust fumes. The peaceful swells of the water become crashing, swirling waves. The peace of God is trespassed upon by the excess of Man.

I had fun, but hubby and I sought the quiet coves where the loud, gas guzzlers were unlikely to venture. As we kayaked, I told him, "The rare spider lilies are blooming on the Catawba River. I so want to kayak to see them, but I can't. The rapids are probably too much for my healing mastectomy. I would be foolish to go now...but they only bloom for two weeks. I guess I can't see them this year."

"There's a nice path along the river where we could walk and see them," he said.

"Could we do that tomorrow?" I asked, hopeful.

"Sure."

Meanwhile, I am torn and must make a decision in the next couple of weeks regarding breast reconstruction Round 2. Do I pay the extra $5k or so out of pocket for the lift of the normal left breast so the two match?

As long as I am going to all the trouble and pain to make the right breast perfect with a nipple, and then tattoo to color the nipple normally, shouldn't I go whole-hog and have the left one not dangle a foot below the level of the right one? (Quit laughing ladies. Wait till you are sixty.)

However, do I really want the extra pain, risk, and expense?

Dr. L wants to do liposuction of my thighs to harvest some fat to fill in the lumps of the right breast. But that adds two new scars and sore healing areas to my already *I've had enough pain for a lifetime* body. I read that silicone implants vs. saline ones will give a smoother appearance to slender women. Will that be enough?

I vacillate daily from one decision to the other. I wonder what will convince me definitively of what I should do.

John 14:27

Peace I leave with you; my peace I give to you. Not as the world gives do I give to you. Let not your hearts be troubled, neither let them be afraid.

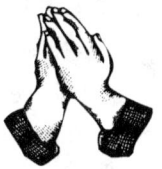

Remembering

May 30, 2016

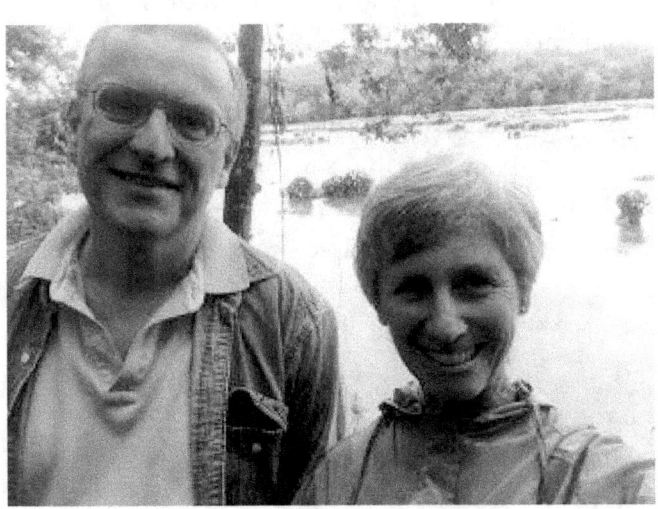

First, on Memorial Day today, I pause and pray with gratitude for those who died for my freedoms. I pray for their families who suffered so much that I might live in a land where I can freely worship and thank God openly. In many places, that is not allowed.

Behind us, in the photo at the top of this blog, is the world's largest stand of rare spider lilies, right on my beloved Catawba river. Last year, I kayaked through those incredible mounds of water-encircled flowers. Yesterday, due to my recent mastectomy, I had to content myself with seeing them from the trail. Navigating the rapids by kayak only four weeks out from surgery would be foolish. They were still breathtaking.

After gazing at the glorious lilies for quite some time, we continued on the Canal Trail, which snaked beside the old Lansford Canal. The remnants of the canal were quite beautiful. It had been raining all morning and threatening to rain more, so the normal crowds that come for the brief blossoming of the lilies were not there. We had the trail largely to ourselves.

When we came home, Lucky had shown us how he felt about us leaving him alone. He had dumped his food bowl, and scattered his food all over the kitchen floor. The past two days, he's done the same thing, only with his water bowl. This is new behavior, and clearly a doggie temper tantrum.

We can't bring him on walks anymore because he is very stiff and goes lame after short walks. I do walk him to the corner of our street and let him sniff and remember the good old days.

I can relate to his angst. I loved seeing the Spider Lilies, but with a tinge of sadness. They only bloom for about two weeks each year. Last year, I kayaked through them with my daughter. I was a little frightened, as there were small rapids the entire way and I am not a whitewater kayaker. My daughter found the rapids tame. She could have just been *acting* cool since that's what teenagers do. Now she's married, and off on her own. I wonder if she remembered that kayak trip through the lilies with the same fondness I do.

As I stood on the trail path yesterday, sidelined by the mastectomy, I looked at the water lilies but remembered the things that are passed now, and will never again be. I understand Lucky's dismay, left behind because he can no longer manage what he loved so much to do.

It is easy to fall into melancholy over what once was, but can no longer be. The Bible warns us that this is not wisdom, to compare the former days with our current situation. Our situations will change, and both the past and present will pass away. Our focus should never settle on the things that were never meant to last forever, but on the One who will. Jesus Christ is the same yesterday, today, and forever. Take comfort in that truth. Let the memories of the past be pleasant, but never a substitute for the true source of delight.

Hopefully next year, all will be well, cancer behind me. The water lilies will bloom again, and God willing, I will kayak in their fragrant midst again. If not, I will remember that He who made the lilies that only flower for two brief weeks, made *me* for eternity. You too!

Ecclesiastes 7:10

Say not, "Why were the former days better than these?" For it is not from wisdom that you ask this.

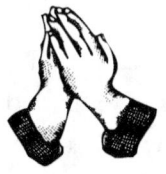

He Will Never Leave Me

May 31, 2016

I love bike riding. I have had to ease slowly back into it since the mastectomy because if I ride too fast, my breathing is deep, and it expands my chest so much that I am in pain. As long as I go slowly, I am fine. This has been a hard lesson for me. I don't like slowing down. However, I have no choice.

On my bike, I was trying to keep up with my husband. I knew I was going too fast for my battered body, but I didn't want to fall so far behind. The sharp pains in my chest got my attention. I stopped and got off my bike. I tried calling to my husband, but he was too far ahead to hear me. Besides, trying to yell hurt more. I rested my head on my handlebar, wondering if this sidewalk, on the side of a busy road would be my final resting place.

If I die here, so be it. At least I will have died doing something I loved. But I'd prefer not to die.

Actually, I knew I wasn't dying, but it *did* hurt. The expander for the breast reconstruction is under the pectoral muscle. When the muscle is further stretched as in extended deep gulps of air, it screams at me. I think it fights the over-stretch by trying to contract. However, it can't because the metal expander prevents that. In a month, the muscle will relax, having become accustomed to the stretch. It will be time to remove the expander and put in the permanent implant. Presumably, I will be able to breathe deeply in exertion without pain again. For now, I didn't move until the pain was gone. The spasm finally passed. From then on, I biked very slowly.

I rarely do too much, or go too fast when I am alone. I listen to my body, and am sensitive to what it is saying. This is why I prefer to kayak, walk, bike, and run alone. God speaks to me, and God never pushes me to go beyond what I am able. God is never disappointed

152

that I am too slow, too fast, or going beyond what someone has advised. God is just there with me. Never too far ahead. Never too far behind. In times of trouble, He is right beside me. If I collapse, He is there to catch me, and tell me it's okay.

I'm here, He whispers through the pain.

He will never leave me nor forsake me. As soon as I accepted Jesus as Lord, His Holy Spirit indwelt me. This miracle is beyond comprehension, but I know it is true. I feel His comfort and guidance from within, deep in my soul, at a place that cannot be shaken.

Anyone going through a serious trial like cancer understands the necessity of a positive outlook. To sustain good cheer for the long haul requires more than just force of character, at least for me. There will always be external forces dragging us down. Always. Anyone who isn't living in a bubble knows this. Whenever I find myself dipping into a trough, I recite scripture, read the Bible, sing songs of praise, pray for others. Invariably this helps remind me I am not alone. No matter what I am going through, Jesus endured worse. And overcame.

He who is in me is greater than the struggle, whatever it may be. This is a promise to those who have entered into a relationship with Christ. I don't rejoice in the struggle, but I rejoice in my God who never abandons me in the struggle.

Deuteronomy 31:8

It is the Lord who goes before you. He will be with you; he will not leave you or forsake you. Do not fear or be dismayed."

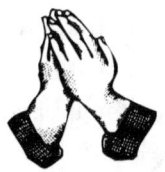

In Quietness and Trust

June 1, 2016

Long bike-ride yesterday on my favorite green-way. I went super slow—nineteen miles in two hours. The Tour de France Bicycle Race is probably not in my future, but I still felt like a champion. Every "normal" activity I can accomplish in the aftermath of the mastectomy a month ago feels like a win!

When I came home, the art demo I had used for my recent art class was still on my easel. It was not very polished. I just draw quickly to guide the class, and then I spend most of my time circulating among the girls and helping them correct their drawings. Sometimes, I just wad up the demo drawing after class, and toss it in the trash.

However, this time, fresh from my bike ride, I looked at the demo picture of an empty path and tree and thought about how I used to pretend my bike was a horse when I was a little girl. I don't *exactly* still do that, but I do feel a connection to my bicycle that isn't *exactly* normal either. For example, I pet it when I dismount.

Does everyone do that? I thought so.

Anyway, the picture of the empty path beckoned me to finish it, to finish it with my dreams. So I drew me in my younger days on a white horse. The book of Revelation in the Bible refers over and over again to a white horse. Jesus Himself will be mounted on the white horse; His name will be "faithful and true." He comes on the white horse to judge in righteousness, and to conquer the forces of evil. Satan and the false prophets will be defeated, thrown (*finally!*) into the lake of fire, and justice will prevail at last.

Wrongs will be righted, evil will be vanquished, and righteousness will reign.

I drew a white horse on the path, my symbol of hope that one day all will be as it should be.

P.S. Today at 10 a.m., I meet finally with my oncologist to go over my treatment plan. My prayer is I will not need chemo or radiation. Please pray for me. *The prayers of the righteous availeth much.*

Revelation 19: 11-20

11 I saw heaven standing open and there before me was a white horse, whose rider is called Faithful and True. With justice he judges and wages war.

12 His eyes are like blazing fire, and on his head are many crowns. He has a name written on him that no one knows but he himself.

13 He is dressed in a robe dipped in blood, and his name is the Word of God.

14 The armies of heaven were following him, riding on white horses and dressed in fine linen, white and clean.

15 Coming out of his mouth is a sharp sword with which to strike down the nations. "He will rule them with an iron scepter." He treads the winepress of the fury of the wrath of God Almighty.

16 On his robe and on his thigh he has this name written: KING OF KINGS AND LORD OF LORDS.

17 And I saw an angel standing in the sun, who cried in a loud voice to all the birds flying in midair, "Come, gather together for the great supper of God,

18 so that you may eat the flesh of kings, generals, and the mighty, of horses and their riders, and the flesh of all people, free and slave, great and small."

19 Then I saw the beast and the kings of the earth and their armies gathered together to wage war against the rider on the horse and his army.

20 But the beast was captured, and with it the false prophet who had performed the signs on its behalf. With these signs he had deluded those who had received the mark of the beast and worshiped its image. The two of them were thrown alive into the fiery lake of burning sulfur.

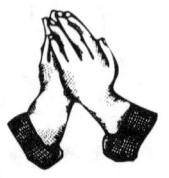

Answered Prayer

June 2, 2016

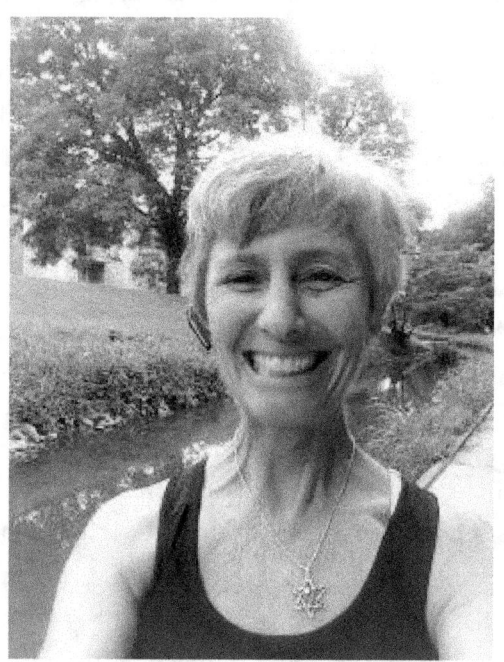

I sat in the oncologist office as the nurse took my blood pressure. 146/82.

"Yikes...that's high for me!"

She nodded.

"I guess I am a little anxious." The nurse didn't comment. Just smiled.

I was indeed anxious. This was the first time I would meet my oncologist, and she had the results of all my tests in her highly trained hands. The onca-type test results had made it into her office late the night before, just in time for my appointment. That would determine how my specific cancer would respond to the medicine, and to chemo. It was critical in directing her advised treatment plan.

I knew a boatload of friends and family were praying for me. I had put out the impossible request. *Please pray for no chemo...and no radiation.*

"It's an audacious prayer," I told one friend.

"May as well pray big!" my friend told me. We do have an audacious God, after all.

The oncologist arrived.

"I hear you are doing really well," she said, after introducing herself. (Hmmm. I wonder who was talking about me.)

"I am. Miraculously really." Cross-shaped earrings dangled from her ears. A believer! Praise God.

"You'll be doing even better when we go over the results."

This boded well!

She was very organized and methodical as she went step by step over all my "numbers." I have perfect estrogen receptors, near perfect progesterone receptors, and excellent Her-2 something or others. Those all weigh in on the risk of recurrence, as well as the response to medicine and to chemo.

I bet my blood pressure was now 197/90...and rising. I tried to read ahead, since she was showing me the chart with all my results, but it was Greek to me.

"Now what this means is you will respond exceedingly well to the medication. The surgeon felt he got all the tumors, but sometimes little microscopic cancer cells can still be there. The medication will get those extremely well, based on your numbers."

200/110 and rising.

Cut to the chase! I didn't say that, but was fidgeting a bit. I could explode right there on the examining table, spewing microscopic bits of cancer everywhere.

"Now," she continued, "I understand you are a big exerciser...I hear you are walking a lot. Studies show that those who exercise at three miles an hour for half an hour five days a week have a significantly lower incidence of recurrence."

"I'm walking eight miles in two hours...eleven miles a day usually," I said. Her eyes opened wide.

"Next, your BMI is at the absolute lowest risk for recurrence." (In other words, skinny is good!)

"Finally, here are your onca results."

210/130 for sure. My eyeballs were probably protruding right out of their sockets. I am sure my pupils were dilated.

"Now four years ago, with four tumors and any lymph nodes involved, we would not be having this discussion. Chemo would be a no-brainer. However, look at this graph of your onca-test."

I looked. I saw a line that started at a place labeled *little risk*, and ended at *high risk*. There was no obvious indication where on that line my onca-test results fell.

"See here? Your first tumor has a score of 1. I have only once seen one score lower. This means there is one percent chance of that cancer returning without chemo. The other tumor, the larger one is a score of 8. Both are extremely low. So low in fact, that you would have a greater risk of the cancer returning *with* chemo."

"Does that mean no chemo?" I said, hardly daring to believe what I thought I was hearing.

"No chemo."

"Praise God!" I shouted, "That is an answer to prayer."

"I thought you'd say that," she said, smiling at me.

"What about radiation? Will that great medicine get all the microscopic cells?"

"Yes...so the radiation is a discussion you need to have with Dr. Bobo."

"I love his name," I told her.

"So do I. He can maybe do very targeted radiation just on the axilla (underarm) lymph area."

"Can we start the meds, and hold off on radiation till after my breast reconstruction?" I asked, "And till after my trip in July to New York to see my siblings and parents?"

"I think that would be fine," she said, "Though you need to meet and discuss that with Dr. Bobo as well."

"Is there a chance I won't need radiation...the medicine will be enough?"

"If it were me, I'd probably get the radiation, but it certainly is worth discussing."

I gripped her hand tightly as she wished me well, and left the room. The nurse hugged me after I checked out. I don't imagine too many happy miracles happen in that building.

After texting all my loved ones, calling my folks, and letting my Facebook prayer warriors know what a glorious result they had been involved in, I headed out to the lovely green-way by the hospital.

I walked to the nearby lake, and meandered along countless paths for seven exultant miles. I think I probably scared some people with my grin as wide as the Atlantic...and I was talking out loud at times. Saying things like: *I can't believe it.* And *Thank you Jesus!* And *Is this really true?*

The picture at the top of this entry is of pure joy. Forgive the selfie...but I wanted to record how powerfully joyful and blessed I felt. I sang loud praises to God, and smiled at everyone I passed.

If God had sent a different result, I was ready to accept it. I had no choice. It was nothing I could control, so I asked God to give me the strength to deal with whatever I had to deal with. I could not believe that what I was dealing with was so *wonderful.* It's been a long time since *wonderful* has smacked me so hard in the face.

No chemo! I can keep my hair, my eyebrows, my eyelashes, my lunch...Such an audacious prayer. Such an audacious God.

Speaking of lunch, I went to Panera's and ordered my favorite salad. I had to celebrate! Plus, those seven miles worked up a powerful appetite. I didn't even mind when the server didn't give me butter for my roll.

I'm going to live!

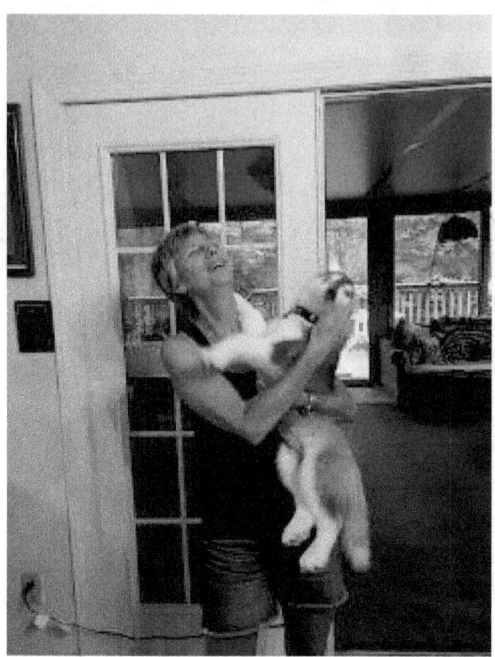

Mark 11:24

Therefore I tell you, whatever you ask in prayer, believe that you have received it, and it will be yours.

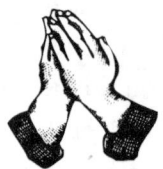

If Only Art were Reality...

June 3, 2016

I had planned to kayak yesterday, but got sidetracked by doing an illustration for a potential new job. The herons at the lake where I kayak had it all to themselves. By the time I finished the detailed illustration, thunder clouds had bloomed and my window of opportunity had closed.

I did learn a very handy new tool on my art program. It is called a lasso. I can choose any part of my drawing, use the lasso tool to encircle it, and then put that section of the drawing anywhere I like. So for example, I lassoed the head of my heron painting, and put the head at its feet.

This is very useful, and I discovered it by accident. There are a million fun things I could do. Endless possibilities! It was almost as much fun as kayaking.

For some reason, this made me think about prayer. I have been on cloud 9 since finding out I don't need chemo and my recurrence cancer risk is very low. But the joy is marred knowing many of my friends *did* need chemo, and some didn't survive cancer. They all prayed for miracles too.

I don't understand. If I had a lasso tool that could lop off tumors and replace them all with strong healthy cells, I would. God doesn't. Not always. I don't pretend to understand. I believe in God's goodness, but I don't understand the pain we endure. Sometimes, I see lessons in the pain and blessings in spite of the pain, but it doesn't lessen the physical anguish. My best attempt at making sense of it all is that this world and all that is in it will pass away. Something more important than our ease and comfort is at stake.

I am so grateful for the blessings I have enjoyed. Last night, as I prayed, I asked that God would give me an ability to see beyond things as they are, to what they one day will be. An eternal perspective is the only way to navigate a world of grief.

Meanwhile, I will lasso despair, and replace it with joy as I have opportunity. It is the best I can do.

Matthew 5:4

"Blessed are those who mourn, for they shall be comforted.

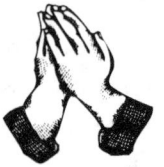

God's Gracious Rewards

June 8, 2016

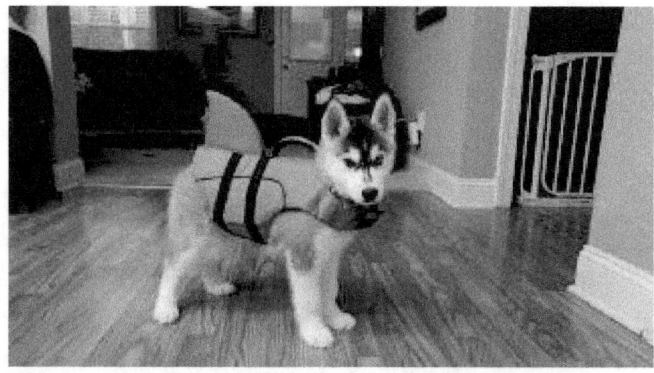

Do you see that adorable "land shark"? That is who I get to spend the next three days with. Well, and my daughter and her new hubby too, but the moment she got a cute puppy, her cuteness was inconsequential. I *love* puppies and this one is especially adorable. My first granddog!

We will be in a cabin in the middle of nowhere along the New River. My birthday gift to my favorite daughter is an all-expense-paid vacation on the banks of the New River, complete with a long horseback riding trip along the New River trail. Our cabin is right on the river, and she was very excited to buy her new pup, Ragnar, a life vest so he can swim in the river.

I am bringing kayaks, my bicycle, and my horse riding boots. This is as close as I suspect I will ever be to heaven on earth.

I am six-weeks post-mastectomy now, and the trauma is but a distant nightmare. I have planned something special each month to look forward to in the midst of the surgeries and treatment. This is my first formal celebration of life and God's goodness. Less formal celebrations occur every moment, as I take in a breath of oxygen and exhale. Miracles of God's love.

I have been told that an essential part of my cancer recovery is to de-stress. I am taking that seriously. (But not *too* seriously, or that would be stressful.) God has opened this exquisite moment for me, and I am seizing it. Living a purposeful life for Jesus is often a hard and arduous path. This does not mean that it should be joyless.

God rewards those who seek Him. I have ardently sought Him, however imperfectly. It has been a very hard road for some time. I wanted to give up more than once. However, no matter how hard it was sometimes to *follow* God, it was always harder *NOT* to follow Him. I am exulting in the reward.

Deuteronomy 28:1-68

"And if you faithfully obey the voice of the Lord your God, being careful to do all his commandments that I command you today, the Lord your God will set you high above all the nations of the earth. And all these blessings shall come upon you and overtake you, if you obey the voice of the Lord your God. Blessed shall you be in the city, and blessed shall you be in the field. Blessed shall be the fruit of your womb and the fruit of your ground and the fruit of your cattle, the increase of your herds and the young of your flock. Blessed shall be your basket and your kneading bowl.

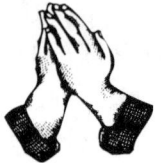

Peace Lighting our Path

June 9, 2016

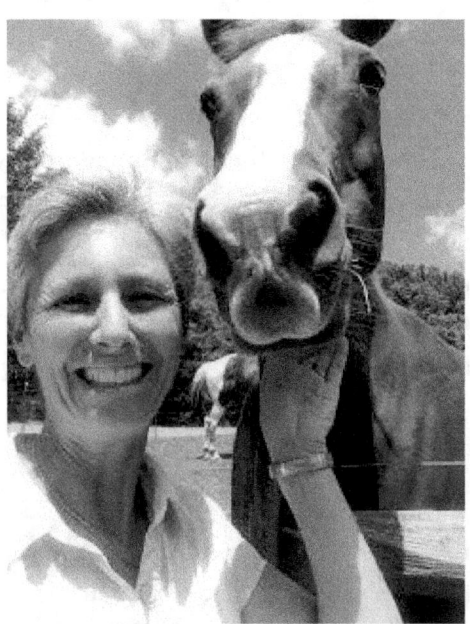

For God to give songs in the night, He must **first** make it night.(Nathaniel William Taylor)

This was quoted in a Bible study my hubby and I did the night before I left for the beautiful New River Trail State Park in Virginia where I am treating my daughter and her new husband to a couple of days of kayaking, swimming, and horseback riding. We are staying in a charming cabin right on the river. This morning we go for our long horseback ride, and then afterwards, will attempt to take their new pup kayaking.

It is stunningly beautiful here. We are nestled between a thickly forested mountain behind us and the gurgling river before us. There is no one else within miles of us. I sat on the porch with my kids last night, watching the river. When Peace like a river attendeth my way.... Those words by the hymnist Horatio Spafford are some of my favorite. The line right after it echoes the quote by Taylor at the top of the blog: When sorrows like sea billows roll. Whatever my lot, Thou hast taught me to say, It is well, it is well with my soul.

The peace...and the sorrow must both exist for one to truly understand the other. Without the night, we cannot learn to sing in the darkness. It is easy to sing with an outpouring of joy to our Lord when all is well, all is lovely, all is just, and all is light. But the world rarely complies.

It has been a long, dark season for me. I don't need to go into details. You can trust me on this. The cancer was just the icing on the cake. There were times I was certain night would never end, morning would never come, the sun would never rise, and peace would never wash over my soul again.

But somehow, even in the midst of all the darkness, peace came. Not in abundance. Only in snatches, at inexplicable moments. It was enough. I understood something I would never have grasped when all was well.

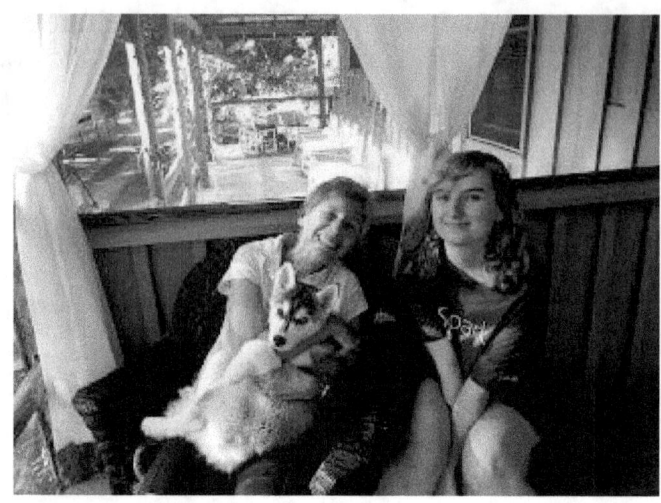

As I counseled a mama a few days ago to choose life over abortion, we talked about God. I asked her if she feared death. She does, like most of us. I asked if she could live forever, would she? She would. Like the long ago seekers of the fountain of youth, that desire is in all of us for permanence, eternity.

"No desire God gives you cannot in some way be fulfilled," I told her, "Or else why would He give you the desire? That would just be cruel. The desire for eternity can be fulfilled. It is fulfilled through Jesus."

Similarly, we hunger, we thirst, we tire, because all those desires can be satisfied. We would not long for peace if peace were not possible.

It is in God alone that we find peace. I wish everyday were littered with beauty like my daughter with her new puppy, the lush mountain and river as a backdrop, tenderness, and love surrounding us all. But the mystery and key of our human existence is to see God when all is not as it should be.

Know He is always there, even when the night is darkest. If you listen to Him, and trust Him, yes, it is possible to sing in the night, but you don't know that till night feels like it will never become light.

One day it will be light again. This is the promise to all who put their hope and faith in Jesus.

Luke 1:77-79

[77] to give knowledge of salvation to his people

in the forgiveness of their sins,

[78] because of the tender mercy of our God,

whereby the sunrise shall visit us[a] from on high

[79] to give light to those who sit in darkness and in the shadow of death,

to guide our feet into the way of peace."

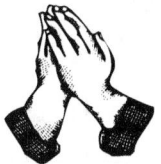

Conquering Darkness

June 11, 2016

I hated to leave paradise. I know how Adam and Eve must have felt.... Our three days at the New River Trail cabin came to an end. I kissed my dear daughter Asherel, her husband Levi, and the adorable husky pup Ragnar goodbye, and they headed home. I still had a whole day before I had to head home. So I first went for a walk as the sun rose. Carl Jung said that in healing one's psyche, it was important to be useful, and to surround oneself in beauty.

Well of course! God never creates without a purpose. The beauty of the world is meant to be inspiring, restorative, and for our enjoyment.

After my walk, I headed to the river with my kayak. The kids had kayaked the day before while I puppy-sat. Now it was *my* turn. I launched, and headed upstream. I really *really* wanted to do the Level Two rapids downstream, but I was very afraid. So I kayaked the smooth water upstream from the launch point. Three Bald Eagles soared over me, completing my bucket list of joyful encounters.

After kayaking about an hour, I came upon small rapids. It was not easy beating upstream to get around them, but I did, which gave me the opportunity to now practice on little rapids.

I made my way quickly back downriver, and came to the take-out point, right before the Level Two rapids. I wanted *so badly* to have the courage to do those rapids...but just *didn't*. I *almost* did, having done the small rapids upstream successfully, but fear overcame me. So I pulled up to shore, about to get out of my boat, when I saw some nearby people in tubes bobbing on the river. They hesitated, and then with a determined shove, shot into the rapids.

Without giving myself time to chicken out, I turned my boat into the current. As the strong current grabbed the boat, there was no turning back. I was now going to do a series of Level Two Rapids, ready or not.

The first set of rapids were very exciting, but not nearly as big as the second set. I was frankly TERRIFIED. I didn't know which path through the frothing water was the best course, and ended up going over a small waterfall. I took on some water, but didn't capsize. On to the next waterfall. More water, but still upright! I finished the rapids, and coasted to the take-out point, exultant, with heart-rate *way over* a sustainable level.

I stood on shore, looking back at the rapids. *I did it!*

I had strapped my kayak cart to the back of the kayak, just in case I somehow mustered the courage to do the rapids. With no one to shuttle me back to my car, I was on my own. Now, I plopped my kayak on the cart, and pulled it the mile back to my car. I could not stop smiling. I had been terrified, and certain this was something I would not dare to do...and then *I did it*. Before I went, I told myself, "If I don't do it now, I may never have another chance...and I might always regret that I didn't have the courage to do what I so wanted to do." I am sure there is a spiritual lesson there.

For one thing, had I not practiced on the smaller rapids, I don't think I would have had the courage to try the larger ones. God sends trials not to confound us, but to prepare us. The more we conquer, the more we learn the power of His presence with us in the midst of the struggle, and the more we trust Him to accomplish the work He has set before us.

I'd been on the water two hours and was ravenous. Fortunately, I had a cooler filled with food which I'd brought to the cabin. Perfect for a picnic in the shade, looking out over the old train that had once traveled the path now made into a biking/hiking trail at this wonderful state park. Carl Jung would have approved. So much restorative beauty.

Having finished my lunch, there was still enough time to go on a final bike-ride. Tossing my picnic trash in the car, I headed off on my folding bike, back down the shady trail flanking the river. I spooked an owl, a skunk, and some woodchucks. The summer crowd has not yet descended and I was almost completely alone on the trail. It gave me lots of time to reflect on God's goodness and the beauty of His creation. I also thought about overcoming fear, and living as if today is the last day you have...because it might be.

I came across many interesting sights, including an old "stone crusher."

By the time I had made it back to the car, I had spent the day logging a four-mile walk, a five-mile kayak, and a seventeen-mile bike ride. As I put the bike in the car, next to the kayaks, I said, "I'm tired."

But it was a *good* tired. A tired that says *every blessed moment of the day God has given me has been used to the fullest.* My batteries are recharged. I am ready again to do battle. I drove home with visions of sweet puppy kisses, my daughter's laughter, frothy rapids in a winding river, soaring eagles, and a bike path speckled with patches of sun beckoning me so strongly that I almost couldn't turn back towards home.

There were messages on my phone. Calls I had missed. There was no cell phone reception at the cabin and so for three days, the outside world vanished for me. There was just me, God's creation, and God. I really hated to leave paradise.

Carl Jung also said, "*When the darkness grows denser, I would penetrate to its very core and ground, and would not rest until amid the pain a light appeared to me, for 'in excessu affectus'* [in an excess of affect or passion] *Nature reverses herself.*"

I don't know what Jung's relationship with Jesus was, but I found his words to be very similar to what Jesus says about light and darkness. Jesus said, *"I am the light of the world. Whoever follows me will not walk in darkness, but will have the light of life."(John 8:12)* The Bible tells us the way out of darkness is to seek the light, and that light is Jesus. Colossians 1:13 tells us *He has delivered us from the domain of darkness.*

The presupposition in all the Biblical verses about light is that you only seek the light after being in darkness.

The people who walked in darkness have seen a great light; those who dwelt in a land of deep darkness, on them has light shined. (Isaiah 9:2)

My thoughts have dwelt for a long time on this, since I am emerging from a very dark tunnel in my life. The only way I made it through the blackness closing in around me was to keep my eyes on the speck of light, of hope at the end of the tunnel.

No one wants to go into the darkness, but it is bearable if we can see light at the other end.

And when we emerge, we are in the light as He is in the light.

...that you may proclaim the excellencies of him who called you out of darkness into his marvelous light.1 Peter 2:9

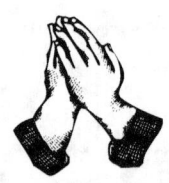

Hard Decisions

June 16, 2016

Decisions are never easy, especially when they can mean the difference between life and death...

I met with my radiologist yesterday to discuss whether radiation is needed or not. The short answer is *yes*, according to him. That is not what I wanted to hear but he certainly painted a *compelling* case.

When I left the appointment, I sat down to try to summarize by writing the *compelling* case, so I could understand, and found I *didn't* understand. I have a call back to him to clarify. Here it is, as I see it. I am certain I am missing something.

My recurrence risk for cancer is 8%. Hormone drug therapy cuts that to 4%. Radiation therapy cuts that by 50% again. I think. Frankly, it was a little confusing. He said because there was lymph involvement, they do radiation to prevent having to do more lymph surgery. He also said that the hormone drug I will be on, which cuts recurrence in half, is *systemic,* but radiation is *local* treatment (targeted on the breast/armpit.) That supposedly also cuts the risk in half. I don't get this, and here is where I drove him and the nurse crazy. If it recurs locally...it still recurs...so who cares if it is systemic or local treatment? With the drug, my risk goes to 4%. Radiation would take it to 2%. If that is the case, I am not sure it is worth going through radiation when my risk is so low...unless I am totally misunderstanding. The nurse who took my call seemed to indicate I was misunderstanding.

I know I am driving my doc and my nurse up the wall. I asked it every way to Sunday, and they didn't seem to understand what I was asking or how to answer my question without ambiguity. I am not being a pain in the neck, at least not *just* because I am a jerk. I don't want to take such a serious decision lightly. Bombarding my body for six-weeks with radiation is a hard thing to dismiss as trivial. If I am not fully behind this treatment, I am sure it will be even less fun than it is already promising to be.

Then, dilemma #2. Ideally, the radiologist starts radiation *now*. But it must go six-weeks uninterrupted. That means, I would have to cancel the trip to see my folks, my sister, and Cape Cod. The best window for radiation is in the first three-months after surgery. So, ideally, I *should* cancel the trip if I decide on radiation. However, the radiologist agreed that quality of life matters, and he understood why I would not want to cancel the trip.

I meet with the surgeon today. My second half of the reconstruction surgery (the easier half I am told) is currently scheduled for August 1, but then that would further push radiation back. The radiologist typically does radiation before the second surgery. So surgery *could* be pushed back, but I must make a decision quickly as the operating room facility fills fast.

So, I am not at all sure what I should do. I am praying about it, and hoping answers will come.

There is a third dilemma too. Right now the reconstructed breast is perky like a 16-year-old's. The normal breast is *obviously* of an old lady pushing six decades of succumbing to gravity. I can get it "adjusted" during the second surgery. However, insurance doesn't pay for it...and it *does* cause a little more pain and suffering.

But, there is *this*. Frankly, it is hard to look in the mirror and feel so freakish. There will be no pictures, so you are going to have to trust me on this.

I went on a long eight-mile walk and prayed. *Show me Lord!* These are not easy decisions, and I really haven't the slightest clue what I should do. I added my 2x4 prayer: *I am thick headed, Lord. You are going to have to smack me over the head with an answer or I won't get it."*

Pray for me if you think of it. I want to do what God would have me do...but I just am not sure what that is.

On a positive note, the little baby saved from abortion, and then born only to have serious respiratory issues had a bad turn two nights ago and went on full oxygen support. However, the mom and many of you prayed all morning yesterday over that sweet little guy. His breathing normalized, and he is now only on 44% oxygen support. Keep the prayers coming, dear friends!

The prayers of a righteous man availeth much.

Philippians 4:6

Do not be anxious about anything, but in everything by prayer and supplication with thanksgiving let your requests be made known to God.

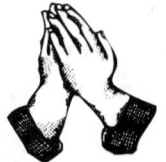

Peace, and Turmoil, Victory and Disappointment: God Sends Them All

June 17, 2016

Well, my oncologist and radiologist made it clear. Radiation is *necessary*. I am very glad that I spent part of the morning kayaking, emptying my mind of all concerns, and felt an hour or so of utter peace. I needed it. It was an emotional day, with a flurry of phone calls, weighing a million pros/cons and cost factors, none of which were easy for me to deal with. I am sorry to report that I cried over the phone a few times. Kind of freaked the hospital business office people out a little... So much for the peace kayaking gave me...

Here's the scoop. The hormone meds which I will take for five years kill cancer cells that may be lurking in my system. The radiation will target any cancer in the lymph nodes, from which new cancer can spread rapidly. Since the surgeon only took out three nodes, and two of them had cancer, rather than rip out *all* my nodes, they radiate the area to kill any cancer that might still be there. Both the meds and radiation are necessary, and both *together* significantly increase my survival rate.

The oncologist didn't pause when I asked her if I should do radiation. She said it was a *must*. Since I really trust her, I am moving forward with that. She is a Christian, and she is very well versed in homeopathic, and natural methods of fighting cancer. She melds them with the medical model. I feel confident on both a spiritual and medical front that she would advise wisely.

When I met with my plastic surgeon later in the afternoon, he told me he wanted to do the second reconstruction surgery before radiation. He said he has a better result when not having to work with radiated skin. However, radiation has to start within three-months of the mastectomy to be most effective. So he scrambled, and in the hour I was there, he consulted with the radiologist and arranged a July 1 surgery. The radiologist agreed that an Aug. 1 start date for radiation is safe. I am just waiting for them to verify they have an operating room available before that date gets chiseled in stone. I should know later today.

I have to miss my NY trip in July...but I will be recovered and done with everything by mid-September and will visit my folks then. Sadly, my health had to take precedence over my desire to travel and see family right now. I feel better having made a firm decision. I felt like God hit me over the head with the direction I needed to go, just like I asked. I didn't love the direction He chose, but I love *Him*...so I will follow.

It was an emotional day. I didn't want radiation, but God doesn't always give us what we want. What He gave me instead was an hour of complete peace while I kayaked, and then firm counsel by people I trust regarding which treatment was necessary. This is often the way He works. He may send disappointment, and tough trials our way, but He never leaves us floundering without someone or something to bolster our spirit and buoy our hope.

Many friends wrote to me with their opinion and advice. I was amazed again by how many people are concerned, involved, and eager to offer love and prayer.

The surgeon told me the drawback to putting the final implant in my breast before radiation is that scar tissue can shrink and tighten the area, and it may become uncomfortable. It might have to even be removed. (If you are keeping count, that would be surgery #3...)

"Well then I will alert my friends to pray that doesn't happen!" I said.

"I hope you have a lot of friends," he said smiling.

"I do."

I feel like every reader, and every Christian who hears of my need is my friend, based on the outpouring of kindness and concern. Thank you friends.

It all helped. I weighed every comment, and let it simmer in my soul. I am disappointed about the radiation...but I am excited to get that second operation over with so soon. I just want the hard stuff behind me!

There was some decidedly good news yesterday as well. Little Baby S who I have been writing about for the past three days took a sharp turn for the better. He is now almost completely breathing on his own, and the mom should be able to finally hold him in the next day or two. Everyone is rejoicing.

I thought about why God might have sent such a severe trial to a mom who had been ready to abort this child at one point. *Why test her further?* In the terrible days when they weren't sure the baby would live, she prayed as she had never prayed before. She also recognized how strong her maternal instincts were, and how all she wanted to do was hold and protect that child. That was probably a good thing for her to realize—the anguish when she thought she might lose him.

Sometimes, I think God teaches and guides us to a higher moral consciousness by showing us glimpses of devastation when we choose to move outside His plan. One cannot know the mind of God, but I wonder if the fragility and sacredness of precious life was what God was conveying in this heart-wrenching time, embedding it firmly in her soul.

The mama could not abide the thought that her baby might die...though it was that very thought that brought her to the abortion center where I met her. I hope and pray she will never return to a place like that again.

John 10:10

The thief cometh not, but for to steal, and to kill, and to destroy: I am come that they might have life, and that they might have [it] more abundantly.

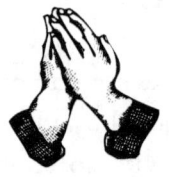

God's Child — Learning About Treasures in the Darkness

June 18, 2016

It's definite. My second phase of reconstruction surgery is July 1, with radiation beginning August 1. As my sister said, "I can think of better ways to spend the summer."

Yes. Only about a *gazillion*...

However, I have learned to say (too many times to count) over the past few months: "It is what it is." I can't change it, and fighting against it only brings me down. I must seek to find the sparks of joy in the midst of the darkness.

Like this: without cancer, I would never have discovered Turmeric Tea. I have come to love it! It is made with several cancer fighting spices, and it is so delicious! I can't say I loved the first sip, but it grows on you. *And, another example:* if sister Amy hadn't come to help me with the first surgery and noticed how our water tasted terribly of chlorine, I would not have gotten my brand new water purifier.

That water is *delicious!* I'd grown so used to drinking terrible water that I didn't even understand what I was missing. I didn't know how good water could be, *should* be! Contemplate that message.

Here's a super-duper blessing. The plastic surgeon insists that to smooth out the appearance of the reconstructed breast he must liposuction my thighs and add fat to the new breast. He reminded me that women pay lots of money for liposuction, but I get it for free, a bonus of this operation. Of all my body parts, my thighs strike me as too large for my otherwise small body. I would never have altered what God gave me if it wasn't necessary. The surgeon says it's necessary.

See? Behind every rain cloud, the sun is still shining.

The mama of Baby S sent me a picture of her holding her little boy for the first time. Their faces reflect joy and serenity. (For privacy reasons, I can't share it.)

"Thank you so much," the grandmother texted me, "Just know what you and the other people that have helped my daughter and other women have done...you all have saved lives of precious little human beings. So worth it. Thank you. And God saved his life not once, but twice. He is God's child."

From the darkness of cancer, I found new healthy ways to live and cope and trust in God. From the darkness of abortion, a mama discovered the deep meaning of sacrificial love. Sometimes it requires a season of darkness to know we are drinking poisoned water and something much, much better awaits us. I am grateful that light dispels the darkness, but even in the darkness there are hidden treasures.

Isaiah 45:3

And I will give thee the treasures of darkness, and hidden riches of secret places, that thou mayest know that I, the LORD, which call thee by name, am the God of Israel.

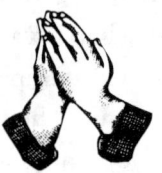

Seizing Opportunity

June 19, 2016

God blessed us with a low humidity, low 80s day. Since I only have two weeks before my second breast reconstruction surgery, I dashed out to kayak. I will not be able to kayak after the surgery for several weeks. Best to seize the opportunity now.

It was perfect kayaking weather. I have not been able to kayak my favorite river because the marina there closed the public launch access. However, I found a park down the street from them, and used my kayak cart to transport my kayak the few hundred feet to the water.

It was wonderful. Much of my time was spent on a creek off of the main river. Some people go a little ways down it, but most turn around before following it very far. I followed it till it was getting too shallow to go much further. It is a little spooky the further you go. It gets narrow, the trees interlace overhead, and you just *know* it is filled with creepy, crawly, slithering creatures.

No one will ever know or find me if one of those creatures kills me. My body will float in my kayak till it decomposes.

Kayaking is mostly peaceful and calming, but back in the secluded winding creek, all alone with primeval forest all around me, I was feeling a little nervous. I started picturing Water Moccasins jumping into my kayak, fangs bared. Next, I envisioned tipping a hornets' nest from an overhanging branch and being stung by a thousand angry insects. Finally, I considered that stray alligators *do* occasionally wander into the Catawba. Hungry, stray alligators.

This is not relaxing.

With that revelation, I headed back to the open waters. The last thing I need in my reduce-stress-to-fight-cancer battle is freaking out over imagined disasters.

My radiologist made a similar point. He told me most people do really well with radiation, especially someone in as good shape as I am. However, he encouraged me to ask whatever I needed to know to be confident in radiation therapy. My attitude and positive outlook are critical factors in the treatment's success.

Attitude. Positive outlook. Where does one find that?

I am not looking forward to surgery or radiation. Frankly, they both scare me. So in my sleepless hours, after applying Essential Oils that induce sleep, I read the Bible. As often happens, my racing thoughts slowed, my worries began to dissipate, and I fell asleep.

I think it had to do with my attitude. God is in control. He knows my terrors, and what I am facing. He has not abandoned me in the past. He will not abandon me now in my moments of greatest need. However, that doesn't mean I am not afraid. I *am* afraid. Some days are worse than others, but there are times when I just want to run away from what I know I have to face.

At times like those, it is best to dwell on verses like this: *Have I not commanded you? Be strong and courageous. Do not be afraid; do not be discouraged, for the LORD your God will be with you wherever you go." Joshua 1:9*

To be strong and courageous is a command! God doesn't command us to do things that come easily and naturally. There would be no need. He commands us to have strength and courage because they are hard. Of course, at the basis of that courage and dispelling of fear is trusting Him. He promises He will be with me *wherever* I go. Through surgery, through radiation, through recovery, through pain, through struggle, through despair.

It was really quite beautiful as I kayaked through the secluded creek back to the river. I even decided to sing out loud since no one was around. I don't know the song very well, but I did remember these words: *"I am not alone. You are always with me, you will never leave me."*

Only God… and the creepy crawly creatures… were listening.

Isaiah 41:10

Fear not, for I am with you; be not dismayed, for I am your God; I will strengthen you, I will help you, I will uphold you with my righteous right hand.

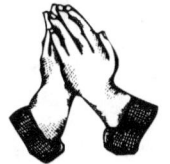

At the End of Yourself, Be Brave in God

June 22, 2016

Before my morning kayak, I got a text from a friend, Cathy. She had been speaking with a young man whose girlfriend was planning to abort the following day. The young man was a friend of her son's and was willing to talk with her, at least a little. However, the young mama would *not* speak to her, and her mind was made up. She would abort. My incredible friend offered the frightened couple her home, money, even adoption of their baby if only they would not abort. They refused.

Cathy encouraged her son and his wife to confront their young, terrified friends. They agreed. Cathy asked me to pray, which I was eager to do. I also gave a whole bunch of advice, based on my experience as a sidewalk counselor at our local abortion center. She asked if her son, Rob, could call me so I could advise him myself.

Of course!

When Rob called, he and his wife put me on speaker phone. They were in the car, en route to meet with the young abortion-minded couple. I talked for an hour, laying out step-by-step what I do in counseling an abortion-minded mama. I gave them an assortment of facts they could use in their discussion. I even sent pictures to their phone of our abortion statistics pamphlet, as well as several websites they should look at before their time with the couple. They took careful notes.

"Remember," I told them, "You are only responsible for being there, for bringing God's message. You are not responsible for the results. That is up to God."

Afterwards, I kayaked on my favorite river, and wondered how this young husband and wife would deal with their first time confronting someone determined to abort. I remembered *my* first time...I was *petrified.* As I skimmed along in my kayak, feeling the peace that always envelops me when I am on the river, I prayed.

Later that day, I received the following text:

Hey everyone. Short update. Our talk went very well. We really got to them, and it got to the point where we pretty much answered everything. It's up to God now.

I could not believe the wisdom coming out of my mouth! God definitely helped us with what we said. Nobody got mad, and we were able to keep the intensity very low and sensitive, and they definitely felt that we were talking to them out of love.

Thank you Vicky for your amazing advice. We wouldn't have been able to do it without you. You will not believe what we just realized! I had taken notes when we were on the phone with Vicky, and right when we started on the subject, I tried to pull them up to refresh myself...but the phone instantly died and wouldn't turn on.

I started to panic, but then I felt like God wanted me to listen to Him, and speak from the heart. And it went really well! My wife just pulled out the phone...and all of a sudden now- it's working and has a decent charge. We didn't plug it in since it died....

God? I think so.

I got chills reading this text. They didn't need their notes or their phone. They didn't need *me*. They could have done it without me. They could *NOT* have done it without God, and they didn't need to.

See, when we are brave in God, and obedient to His call, He empowers us.

There is nothing more exciting than feeling the Holy Spirit take over and bring us to places we know we could not possibly arrive on our own. These obedient messengers of truth to the hurting, abortion-minded couple are *eighteen-years-old*. They have no training in counseling abortion-minded mothers. All they have is a conviction of right and wrong, a desire to heed God's call, and the obedience to be in a place that is terrifying and outside their knowledge and ability.

We don't know what the young abortion-minded couple will choose to do. We don't yet know if their baby will be saved. What I *do* know for sure is that another young couple has just been irrevocably changed, finding a strength and a purpose to their lives that perhaps they had never known they had.

Be brave in God. When you come to the end of yourself, He is ready and waiting. It will amaze you what He can do with a fearful but willing heart.

Deuteronomy 31:6

Be strong and courageous. Do not fear or be in dread of them, for it is the Lord your God who goes with you. He will not leave you or forsake you."

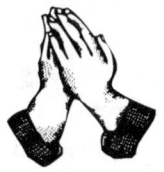

Is My God Big Enough?

June 25, 2016

On a recent run, I was going at a moderate pace. I wasn't planning to run for very long because it was so hot outside. However, by the time I hit mile 4.2, I started feeling good. I kicked into high gear, thinking I will just run fast to the corner.

I pulled out my handy fitness app, *Map My Run,* and saw I was doing a 7:15/mile pace. I was sure it was a mistake. I haven't run that fast since I was twenty. So, suddenly, I was on a mission. Could I maintain that pace for two miles to finish out a 10K?

I was running *for sure* to my utmost. Don't think I wasn't gasping for air. I was. However, I was determined to run faster than I thought I could bear. That seemed like something worthwhile to do. I kept the timer in my hand, checking my pace. *I can do this! No, I can't! Yes, I can!*

My second (and last) breast reconstruction surgery is in one week, July 1. I have been told this operation is a breeze as regards to the breasts. HOWEVER, to smooth and perfect the reconstruction, the surgeon will be sucking fat out of my thighs to smooth and pad the new breast.

Friends and the internet seem to concur that the aftermath of this liposuction is pretty terribly painful. I am downright terrified. It is hard to keep my eyes on Jesus when everyone is telling me my eyeballs will be rolling out of their sockets in misery.

I can do this! No I can't! Yes, I can...can I?

Please pray friends. Prayer moves mountains. Pray the pain is bearable, and there are no complications. I will call the surgeon this week to be sure he feels it is absolutely necessary we do the liposuction but I already know the answer. He has already told me the breast reconstruction is better with the liposuction.

I watched my phone click off the mileage, and as soon as it hit 6.2 miles, the distance of a 10k, I clicked *finish* on "Map My Run." The last two miles I averaged below 7:30/mile. *I did it.* I don't know what reserve all that speed came out of, but it showed me something I needed to see.

We defeat ourselves. We are almost always capable of doing more than we believe we are capable of doing. Similarly, we defeat God's work in our lives. Our vision of God is rarely too big...it is usually too small. Can God handle even this liposuction? Of course He can. Can He empower *me* to handle it? Is God big enough for even *this*?

You may not be facing cancer, but I bet you have asked this of God at some point in your life about some overwhelming obstacle. If you haven't, you probably will.

Most of us have some concept of God, and usually it is narrowed by our own limited perspective and experience. A classic book by JB Phillips (*Your God is Too Small*) says we limit God, envisioning him as policeman, conscience, parental voice, a grand old man, meek and mild, or in a box we construct based on our expectations, to name a few titles we give Him. None of those convey the grandeur, power, and awe that God deserves.

Colossians 1:16 tells us that He created all things, the entire universe. Isaiah 45:7 reminds us He formed light and created darkness; He makes well-being and calamity. He numbers and names every star, as well as every hair on our head. No sparrow falls to the ground without his notice. His Providence stretches wider than the universe and as small as numbering our every hair. Who is like Him other than He? Majestic in holiness, awesome in power, eternal... and yet inexplicably concerned with the comparatively minuscule affairs of humankind.

This God can do all things. My friend prayed for me yesterday and told me she was praying I would replace worry with worship. *Yes!* My God is big enough for everything I face. Is yours?

∞

Exodus 15:11

"Who is like you, O Lord, among the gods? Who is like you, majestic in holiness, awesome in glorious deeds, doing wonders?

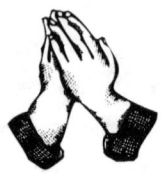

The Right Kind of Fear

June 26, 2016

I got lost on my morning bike ride looking for Caribou Coffee. That's okay. It was a beautiful morning, and I discovered a little creek hidden alongside a secluded path I had never seen before. What a happy surprise! Mapquest helped me find the Caribou Coffee.

I biked home and headed off immediately to kayak. I know. Rest isn't really in my vocabulary. Also, I only have a week till my surgery, and then radiation. I need to cram in as much fun as I can since I don't know if I will be able to do much over the summer with all those fun medical interventions.

Besides, truth be told, I am afraid of my upcoming ordeals. If I stay active in places of beauty and peace, the fear subsides.

I unloaded my kayak at the Catawba riverside park, and was wheeling it on its little cart to the river. A couple of women passed me and one said, "Don't get wet. There's flesh eating bacteria in there."

I thought she was referring to the brain-eating amoeba, which recently killed a girl who was rafting at the nearby Whitewater Center. I knew the amoeba could only reach the brain by being sucked in through the nose. I was in no danger since all I would do was step into the water.

"I won't snort the water," I promised.

"No, not the *amoeba*," the lady said, "Flesh eating *bacteria*. Some kids that were swimming right there..." She pointed to the exact point where I launch my kayak. "...came down with rashes, and were quarantined. It was in the news, though I haven't heard updates. They said it was flesh-eating bacteria."

I had NOT heard about this. I decided since I had other bodies of water I could kayak in, I would instead drive a half hour to Lake Wylie. As far as I know, no flesh-eating bacteria have been reported there.

I thanked the ladies, and drove to Lake Wylie. I was glad I did. It was relatively calm for a Saturday without too many noisy motorboats, and the water felt wonderful. I don't know what I would have done if I didn't have options. Brave flesh eating bacteria or forgo one of my favorite activities on earth?

There are a lot of dangers in the world. The miracle is that most of us do survive through adulthood.

It would be very easy to succumb to fear. There really are a bizarre number of things to be afraid of. Fear could quickly become the motivator for all our activity, and I suspect would reduce our lives to nothing.

The Bible warns us that we who love God should not fear. If we trust Him, we have nothing to fear. This does not mean we should abandon common sense, but a life spent huddled in our closet because so many things out there can kill us is not a life.

Listen to what the Bible says about fear:

Fear not, for I am with you; be not dismayed, for I am your God; I will strengthen you, I will help you, Isaiah 41:10

For God gave us a spirit not of fear but of power and love and self-control. 2 Timothy 1:7

There is no fear in love, but perfect love casts out fear. For fear has to do with punishment, and whoever fears has not been perfected in love. 1 John 4:18

Even though I walk through the valley of the shadow of death, I will fear no evil, for you are with me Psalm 23:4

The fear of man lays a snare, but whoever trusts in the Lord is safe. Proverbs 29:25

For you did not receive the spirit of slavery to fall back into fear, but you have received the Spirit of adoption as sons, by whom we cry, "Abba! Father!" Romans 8:15

The fear of the Lord leads to life, and whoever has it rests satisfied; he will not be visited by harm. Proverbs 19:23

The fear of the Lord is the beginning of wisdom... Psalm 111:10

The message is clear. We should fear nothing on earth. We are only to fear the One who controls all things. He who directs the universe directs our paths. He alone should be the object of fear, since our future is in His hands. A *holy fear* should direct us to follow, cling to, and obey Him, not to avoid catastrophe, but because of the immensity of our love for Him and understanding of His love for us.

This is wisdom, and ironically, this type of fear leads to life. Eternal life.

There are no flesh-eating bacteria in heaven.

Psalm 23:1-6

A Psalm of David. The Lord is my shepherd; I shall not want. He makes me lie down in green pastures. He leads me beside still waters. He restores my soul. He leads me in paths of righteousness for his name's sake. Even though I walk through the valley of the shadow of death, I will fear no evil, for you are with me; your rod and your staff, they comfort me. You prepare a table before me in the presence of my enemies; you anoint my head with oil; my cup overflows.

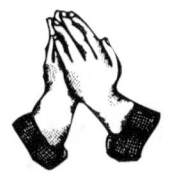

Regard Self Less, God More....

June 29, 2016

I spent much of the day yesterday cleaning the house in preparation for my upcoming surgery July 1. I won't be able to clean for at least a couple of weeks after surgery, so decided I needed to get everything done now while I am still strong and able. I did the laundry, made two loaves of my home-ground healthy bread, vacuumed, dusted, cleaned the bathrooms, mopped the floors, and packed my hospital bag.

To avoid the recurrence of blood clots which I had with the original surgery, I bought rainbow striped compression socks. How fun is that! I was also told I need compression shorts for a couple of weeks for my liposuctioned thighs (they are harvesting fat to aid in the breast reconstruction.) Since I just don't think a near 60-year-old lady should be seen in public in compression shorts, I got some with a skirt over them. *How cute will I be in rainbow knee socks and a little skort with compression shorts?* I will be the talk of the recovery room.

I spent a great deal of time walking and in prayer. As the surgery looms, I find I must constantly be talking to God, or my freak-out potential increases. Charles Spurgeon agrees this is a good strategy. Here is what he said in my morning Bible study:

It is ever the Holy Spirit's work to turn our eyes away from self to Jesus; but Satan's work is just the opposite of this, for he is constantly trying to make us regard ourselves instead of Christ.

I had always thought of this as a call to glorify God rather than self...and of course, it is. But it is *also* protective! When I am facing something terribly frightening or difficult, like the surgery, focusing on myself makes it a thousand times worse. When I focus on Christ instead, the hours pass and I barely consider the upcoming ordeal.

In fact, I am almost *excited* about surgery since I get to wear those rainbow socks. Almost but not quite. In the *not quite* moments, I am focusing on Christ to get me through.

Colossians 3:2

Set your minds on things that are above, not on things that are on earth.

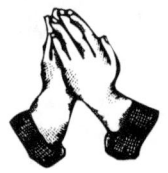

Tranquil waters in Troubled World

June 30, 2016

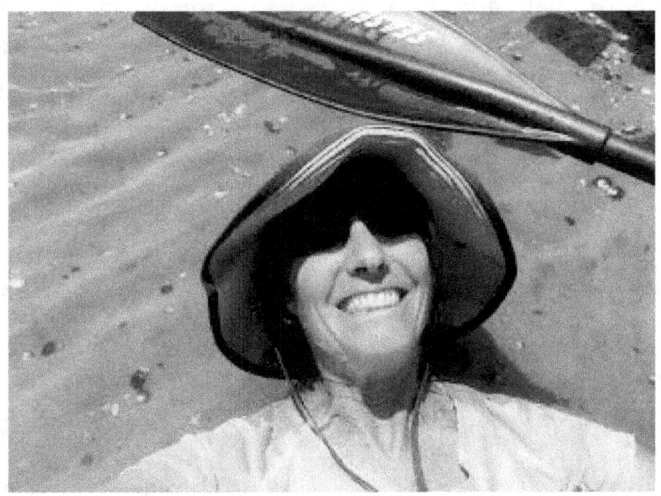

I am lying in Lake Wylie here, though it is kind of hard to tell. There is a little island that I kayak to, where I get out of my boat, lie down in the water, and cool off. Ahhhh! Peaceful waters all around me; the troubled world far in the distance. There is almost nothing as soothing as cool, still waters when you are hot, and tired.

I went kayaking right after getting a bone density scan. That was the absolute least invasive medical procedure I have had to have in a long time! It doesn't hurt AT ALL. The oncologist wanted to see how much calcium had leached from my bones over the years since I already have borderline bone mass and the cancer drug will eat my bones even more. If only everything I faced was so painless....

My plastic surgeon tells me the operation Friday will very likely NOT be my last one. After radiation, the implant for mastectomy breast reconstruction tends to shrink and harden, and many women have to have a third surgery to correct the "capsular contractions". I am NOT LOVING this process.

The radiologist who was on-call for my vacationing doctor went to a lot of trouble to search for some articles that answered my worried questions. He emailed me the research report. The statistics are not encouraging. With the type of reconstruction I have and the surgery tomorrow (which I thought would be the last one), the majority of women who have radiation *after* the reconstruction (like me) will end up with another surgery to fix the effects of radiation. If I wait and have the reconstruction surgery *after* radiation, the reconstruction I have is often unsuccessful or with unsatisfactory results due to the condition of the radiated skin. There is no *good* option open to me, except prayer.

This is never ending! I had no idea when I started this journey how much struggle it would entail, nor how many impossible decisions would have to be made. I have no choice at this point, being half-way through the process, so I spent a lot of time talking to God. *Please Lord, let me defy the odds and have no complications and let this be the last surgery I will need.* I would calm during my chats with Him, and especially when I focused on praying for others, but it was a constant battle to keep my mind focused on God, rather than on my troubled thoughts.

What I am going through is difficult, but we *all* face troubling issues in life. None of us know what we will face when we crawl out of the womb. If we did, we would all crawl right back in. We are often faced with impossible choices, none of which seem perfect or even pleasant. None of us are guaranteed an easy go of it. Truthfully, the Bible says all of us *are* guaranteed times of struggle.

How are we to survive then? Or even better, how do we *thrive* in the midst of this guaranteed pain and suffering? Is kayaking all day every day the only way to find peace? (It works for me to a point...and then my arms give out.)

"Peace be with you." (John 20:19) The promise and hope in the words of the risen Christ are the only peace that will confront and vanquish the terrors of the Enemy.

Fortunately, the lake and kayak worked their magic. My pulse and blood pressure returned to a normal range following the peaceful emptying of my mind before God in the glory of His creation.

Besides, I got two pieces of good news. The baby of one of the mamas I work with who had been in the Neonatal ICU for ten days IS HOME!!!!! Next, the mama who chose life Monday but is still wavering texted me. Her baby is still safe in her womb, and she sounds like she is leaning towards letting him remain there.

So don't feel bad for me. *I am blessed.* Everyone is who has God on their side. Troubles will not cease, but God does provide tranquil water in the midst of this troubled world. Its name is Jesus.

James 1:12

Blessed is the man who remains steadfast under trial, for when he has stood the test he will receive the crown of life, which God has promised to those who love him.

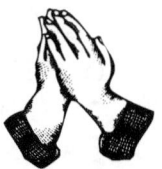

Wait for Him; He will Surely Come

July 1, 2016

Heigh-ho,

Heigh-ho,

To surgery I go!

I received a text from one of the mama's I work with yesterday. She had no idea how much she was ministering to me on the eve before my second breast reconstruction surgery. She had chosen life over abortion several weeks ago, and then experienced terribly dangerous placenta problems. She texted me telling me the placenta had healed itself.

"Were the doctors astounded?" I asked. "Did you tell them WHO healed you?"

Here is her answer:

YES. THEY SMILED ♡ MY PLACENTA WAS COVERING UP MY CERVIX BAD. IF IT WAS TO BUST, I WOULD BLEED TO DEATH. ME AND THE BABY COULD HAD DIED ... THEY WERE GOING TO HAVE TO DO AN EMERGENCY SURGERY BUT WHEN I WENT BACK TO GO DO THAT, FIRST THEY DID AN ULTRASOUND. THEY COULDN'T BELIEVE THE PLACENTA MOVED ON ITS OWN :)))))))) MY BABY IS A STRONG HUMAN BEING. ALL MY BABIES R ♡ VICKY, U DON'T UNDERSTAND HOW U CHANGED MY LIFE IN THE WAY TO THINK WHEN I MET YOU, AND U STOPPED ME FROM MAKING THE BIGGEST MISTAKE IN MY LIFE. I'VE ALWAYS WANTED A SISTER AND NOW MY DAUGHTER WILL HAVE ONE! IMAGINE THAT I WAS GOING TO DESTROY A BEAUTIFUL ANGEL

194

IN MY BABY GIRL THAT I WANTED SO BADDDDD, BUT FELT HOPELESS!! GOD HAS ALWAYS BEEN ON TIME.

As I go into surgery today, that mama's faith, joy, and trust in God will echo in my heart. *God has always been on time.*

I appreciate all your prayers so much. I am confident that God has me in His hands.

Habakkuk 2:3

For still the vision awaits its appointed time; it hastens to the end—it will not lie. If it seems slow, wait for it; it will surely come; it will not delay.

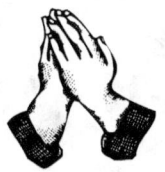

He Spared Me from the Pit

July 2, 2016

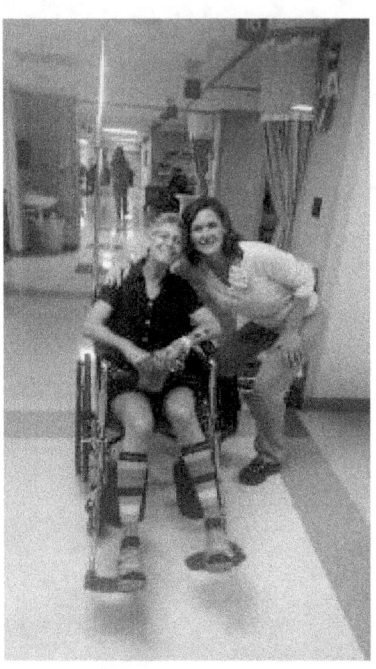

You, Lord, brought me up from the realm of the dead; you spared me from going down to the pit. Psalm 30:3

God is amazing. I was barely conscious in the recovery room, and fighting nausea when my nurse came into focus. It looked like she'd been trying to talk to me a while, and I'd been dodging wakefulness.

"Vicky?" she said. "Remember me....I'm..."

"Sharon!!" we said together.

Sharon goes to my church! I used to teach her kids in my art class! A *friend* had been assigned to be my recovery nurse unbeknownst to either of us!

The surgery day did not dawn so cheerily. I had been up the entire night before surgery with an incredibly painful neck and chest pains. I had a "crick" in my neck for three days, and when I kayaked the last time, it was slightly painful as I made my way back to the dock. Was that the cause of the chest pains now?

I must have badly strained my intercostal muscles because the pain was very bad. I could barely move. I didn't sleep at all. I was pretty sure it wasn't a heart attack, though not certain. I sat upright all night, as it hurt less that way, and read my Bible.

What about the surgery? If it was postponed, the delicate optimal time-frame for radiation would be thrown off. Hubby prayed with me, then drove me to pre-op. The nurse checked me in early, and there was concern I should go to the ER, and forego the surgery.

Fortunately, I was pretty sure it was muscular, and not a heart attack. By the incredible grace of God, the anesthesiologist was a kayaker. When I told him my story, he was very sure it was the intercostal muscles, and not a heart attack. He had experienced the same issue himself! My plastic surgeon arrived, and concurred, but ordered an EKG to be on the safe side. All was normal.

I can't tell you how lovely it was to be knocked out on heavy narcotics for the next several hours for my surgery. I had been in fairly severe pain the entire previous night. As I was struggling all night in pain, I am afraid I succumbed to asking God, "Why??"

Now, on the other side of the surgery, I think I know. I was so sidetracked by the pain of the intercostal muscles that I never worried about undergoing surgery. In fact, I *wanted* the surgery to get me out of such pain! I had been hovering near panic about the upcoming surgery but that was totally eliminated.

I have been pain-free all night and into this morning. There is some soreness in my thighs from the liposuction, but only a feeling of slight bruising. Nothing hurts the way I thought it would. I took one-third of one dose of the narcotic pain-killer last night, and just a tylenol this morn. Sister Amy wants me to stay ahead of the pain, so I did that although nothing hurt.

Since I am to wear the compression socks and shorts for two to three weeks or longer, 24 hours a day to reduce swelling and chance of clots, I ordered one more pair of each online. They are pricey, but worth it.

God always astounds me. What often feels like a disaster ends up a blessing. I am so relieved to be through this surgery. My reconstructed breast looks great and when I looked in the mirror this morning, I smiled. Except for the scars and no nipple...I look normal! To top off that joy, Sharon, my nurse friend was an unexpected and miraculous intervention by my precious Lord.

The portion of the Bible I was reading all night was my favorite story of Elijah defeating the evil prophets of the false God, Baal. When Elijah (with God's help) completes this impossible task, he loses heart and falls into a depressive funk. He feels all alone, and knows a bounty is on his head from the evil Queen Jezebel. He cries out to God to just kill him now. It is too much. He wants to die.

God shows up, provides shade, food, drink, and restorative sleep. Then he comforts Elijah further by telling him he is not alone. He is sending friends.

As I awoke from all the trauma and fear to my friend Sharon's face, I felt the unequivocal miraculous presence of God.

God is so good.

<u>1 Kings 19: 11-18</u>

Then He said, "Go out, and stand on the mountain before the LORD." And behold, the LORD passed by, and a great and strong wind tore into the mountains and broke the rocks in pieces before the LORD, *but* the LORD *was* not in the wind; and after the wind an earthquake, *but* the LORD *was* not in the earthquake; [12] and after the earthquake a fire, *but* the LORD *was* not in the fire; and after the fire a still small voice.

¹³ So it was, when Elijah heard *it,* that he wrapped his face in his mantle and went out and stood in the entrance of the cave. Suddenly a voice *came* to him, and said, "What are you doing here, Elijah?"

¹⁴ And he said, "I have been very zealous for the LORD God of hosts; because the children of Israel have forsaken Your covenant, torn down Your altars, and killed Your prophets with the sword. I alone am left; and they seek to take my life."

¹⁵ Then the LORD said to him: "Go, return on your way to the Wilderness of Damascus; and when you arrive, anoint Hazael *as* king over Syria. ¹⁶ Also you shall anoint Jehu the son of Nimshi *as* king over Israel. And Elisha the son of Shaphat of Abel Meholah you shall anoint *as* prophet in your place. ¹⁷ It shall be *that* whoever escapes the sword of Hazael, Jehu will kill; and whoever escapes the sword of Jehu, Elisha will kill. ¹⁸ Yet I have reserved seven thousand in Israel, all whose knees have not bowed to Baal, and every mouth that has not kissed him."

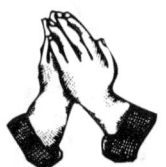

Training Self Physically and Spiritually

July 3, 2016

I am ready to tear up the streets in my compression anti-clot, anti-swelling garb. Since I also have a mouth-drying anti-nausea patch behind my ear, I need to wear my beltpack with a water bottle pouch.

I bet all the neighbors are peeking from behind their curtains, wondering if the surgeons removed more than just my breast.

I went on three separate walks, totaling four miles. Not bad for one day after major surgery! My liposuctioned thighs, harvested of their fat for new duties in my reconstructed breast hurt unless I stay active. After my two hour nap, standing up was not for the faint of heart. But within a minute of walking around, the pain dissipates.

Strange that the more I use the body parts that are healing, the better I feel. This fact is true in physical healing *and* in spiritual healing. All of us are damaged spiritually. All of us sin, and in doing so, slam the door on a proper relationship with God. The only path to healing is first sorrow over how we have grieved God, and then to use our body and mind vigorously in step with Him. Our eyes should be constantly seeking Him, our lips constantly speaking of Him, our ears constantly listening to His word, and our steps following Him. Only then does the pain of our separation from Him dissipate and healing begins.

I never expected to feel this good one day from major surgery!

1 Timothy 4:8

For while bodily training is of some value, godliness is of value in every way, as it holds promise for the present life and also for the life to come.

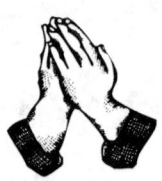

To His Glory

July 4, 2016

While I feel relatively great following my second phase of breast reconstruction surgery, there is only so much healing one can do in a day. Some things we can't speed up, much as we'd like. I do three walks a day, but then crash on the recliner, and nap often in between those walks.

A neighbor, who didn't know I'd just had surgery said, "I noticed you are moving slower than usual."

"I just had surgery," I explained. "I'm not supposed to raise my heart rate."

"Ah. You be careful," he said kindly. I saw him surreptitiously watching me as I shuffled around the block. I think my bright knee-socks in 100 degree heat baffled him.

I moved slowly from shady spot to shady spot. Only very small portions of my walk need to be in the hot, direct sun. It was a little frustrating being unable to walk at a faster pace. I don't slow down easily. However, I want to heal and so I am being very careful to follow doc's orders.

Since I only have one set of compression shorts and socks, I have been wearing the same outlandish outfit the past three days. Bright rainbow knee-socks, with my blue shimmery sandals, and compression shorts with a modest skirt over them. It is a blistering hot season in NC. No one wears knee-socks in 100 degree heat. Except me.

Fortunately, Tuesday a second pair of shorts and socks arrive. I have to wear this compression get-up for a few weeks. Fun!

The nurse assistant who wheeled me down to my car following surgery overheard me talking with my nurse about art classes I teach.

"I *thought* you were an artist!" the assistant said as she pushed the wheelchair down the corridor.

We both glanced at my rainbow socks. I wonder what tipped her off?

Although recovery is going well, there are hard times. Like after I have rested in my recliner and try to stand again, the pain in my thighs nearly fells me. For the first few steps, it is pretty terrible, but then, the hurt subsides. The doctor told me walking was the key to overcoming the swelling and pain in my thighs. Still, it takes a lot of strong talking to myself to get me to move from my painless lounging to a much less painless standing position. I know what I am about to endure, however briefly, and it would be much easier to just stay comfy and pain-free in my recliner.

So guess what that made me think about?

Sometimes we get too comfortable in our Christian walk. We do the basics, read a little Bible, pray a little, and go to church and even stay awake sometimes. However, are we following the treatment plan God has given us for a sick and broken world? Are we going and making disciples, are we glorifying God in our family, our work, our neighborhood? Are we visiting the sick, those in prisons, the widows, and the hungry? Are we sacrificially meeting the needs of those less fortunate than we? Are we protecting the innocent and the vulnerable?

It takes a lot of strength to overcome complacency, stand, and then walk where God is telling us to go. It often *does* hurt...at first. It is unfamiliar, uncomfortable, and painfully awkward. However, I think there is no question that if we are resting in the Lord but not serving Him, we probably will not impact the world to His glory, and our own healing in God will stagnate.

I'd write more about this, but I need to put my full energy into talking myself into standing up now.

1 Samuel 12:24

Only fear the Lord and serve him faithfully with all your heart. For consider what great things he has done for you.

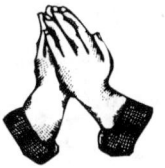

Rejoice Always

July 5, 2016

My second set of post-breast-surgery compression socks arrived yesterday. I had thought they were a southwestern scene, cactus...sun...but my sister Wendy pointed out the images were of a fork with bacon and eggs.

Oh. I still really like the colors...

Meanwhile, gazing at my socks, I noticed my knees had disappeared. There ARE knees somewhere under all that swelling. What is happening to my knees is also happening to my waist and midsection. My waist was gone yesterday. Totally enveloped in swelling. I did call the doc to be sure this is all okay. He said it is normal.

Anyone who would do liposuction by choice is NUTS in my opinion. My chest area, the focal point of all this surgery, barely hurts at all. The liposuctioned thighs are a *totally* different matter.

My body made it clear to me that I needed to rest. I took two naps before lunchtime and two more after. Then I went to bed. I never nap. Liposuction changed all that. Since the only antidote to all the swelling and pain is to walk, I forced myself through the first minute of torture and walked two miles in the morning. Then I was in my recliner napping, and surveying my vanished knees and my ham-and-egg kneesocks until walk #2 in the blistering heat. I was too weak, nauseous, and tired for walk #3. Anyone who knows me knows if I forego a walk, something is wrong.

There are some positive developments. Lately, as I stand up after resting, the searing pain is not so searing. My slight nausea has subsided at least for now. (I did take an anti-nausea pill last night.) My walking pace, despite feeling so badly yesterday, went from 30-minute miles to 21-minute miles. The slight wobbly, unsteadiness as I walk is mostly gone away. The icky drainage tube has collected the minimum yuck from the surgical site, and I will call the doc this morn. I think he will take it out today. (Praise God—the drainage tube is the pits.) My daughter is coming to keep another set of eyes on me and to drive me to doctor if needed. My waist is slowly returning and I can see my kneecaps again. There is progress and cause for rejoicing!

I read a quote on Facebook: *If you are always complaining that your glass is half empty, get a smaller glass, fill it, and stop complaining.*

I like that. Whatever you are handed in life, make it a blessing. Look for the blessing, the positive, the hand of God teaching, comforting, refining, and preparing. The section I read yesterday morning in my Bible study was about Paul imprisoned for two years for crimes he didn't commit. Instead of complaining or railing against the injustice of it all, he proclaimed the Gospel from his jail cell. And he wrote several of the books in the Bible from jail! How many people came to a saving faith in Jesus because Paul chose converting over complaining?

Do you feel like complaining? Listen to what the unjustly imprisoned Paul wrote from prison:

[12] Now I want you to know, brothers and sisters, that what has happened to me has actually served to advance the gospel. [13] As a result, it has become clear

throughout the whole palace guard and to everyone else that I am in chains for Christ. [14] And because of my chains, most of the brothers and sisters have become confident in the Lord and dare all the more to proclaim the gospel without fear.

[15] It is true that some preach Christ out of envy and rivalry, but others out of goodwill. [16] The latter do so out of love, knowing that I am put here for the defense of the gospel. [17] The former preach Christ out of selfish ambition, not sincerely, supposing that they can stir up trouble for me while I am in chains. [18] But what does it matter? The important thing is that in every way, whether from false motives or true, Christ is preached. And because of this I rejoice.

Yes, and I will continue to rejoice (Philippians 1: 12-18)

It was an excellent study for me to read, as I watched my thighs slowly blow up into bloated sausages. Rejoice in the Lord always!

Philippians 2:14

Do all things without grumbling or questioning,

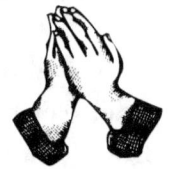

On the Other Side of Despair

July 6, 2016

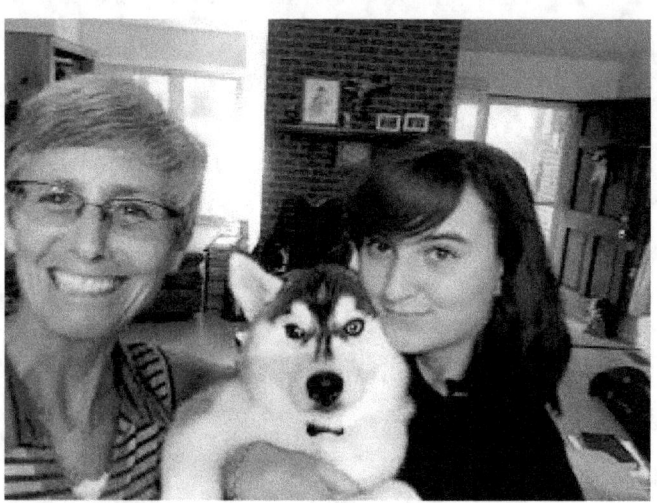

It was a day of joyous surprises on the recovery from my second mastectomy surgery. My beautiful daughter came in the morning to spend the day with me, since I would otherwise be alone and had had a really rough day the prior day. As it turns out, I didn't feel awful, other than lingering nausea.

She came with me to see my doctor who, joy of joys, removed my drainage tube! Major feel good event! Then he told me I didn't have to wear the compression knee-socks anymore! Now, I *will* use those adorable compression socks with their fun colors to run in as they are very good for runners, but what a joy to be able to ditch them in the 100-degree heat wave!

The nurse told me I need to take the anti-nausea meds once a day. Nausea is very common in this surgery, and it would be best to control it. So I did and felt instantly better. With all that good news from the doc, my daughter and I celebrated with Chick-fil-A. I have been very careful to eat only a cancer-fighting prescribed diet, but my oncologist told me it was ok to cheat now and then. So I got fries. Yum.

Bonus: Asherel's adorable dog, Ragnar, spent the day with us as well. I took him on two of my shorter walks. He is the best trained four-month-old puppy I know. He is also very friendly. When a dog passed us by without stopping to say hello, Ragnar sat down and wistfully watched the dog walk away. He would not pay any attention to my tugs on the leash till the dog was out of sight. With a sigh, he turned and followed me home.

I have had a rough time the past couple of years. It went from bad to worse with the breast cancer diagnosis. I didn't handle the despair well in the beginning. I almost lost my sanity wallowing in how the burdens upon me were far beyond my ability to bear.

Then slowly, far too slowly, I began to notice God. Sparks of light in my darkness reminded me He had not left me. They were sometimes little things. Sometimes they were big things, like incredible numbers of mamas choosing life at the abortion center where I volunteer on the sidewalks.

If God is blessing that endeavor, then surely He has not abandoned me!

Despite being certain I could not survive all the terrible things happening to me, I *did* survive. It was clear that *Someone* was shoring me up, holding my arms when I could not lift them on my own.

One of my favorite images in the Bible is of Moses, with the staff of God in his hands, when he is told to fight Israel's enemies. Moses stood atop a mountain overlooking the battle. As long as Moses held up his arms, Israel was winning. When his arms tired and dropped, Israel was losing. His friends, Aaron and Hur came to the rescue and held up Moses' hands. A friend stood on each side of him, while Moses clutched the staff of God tightly. Victory was secured with God and the help of friends.

This is the picture of how I survived. My hands and my heart were raised to God, but there were many times I grew too weary and too overcome to continue. I often lost hope. Friends and family came alongside me and helped hold me up when I was ready to collapse in defeat.

So now, I have finished the last major surgery of my cancer career. (I hope.) I am recovering beautifully. I walked five miles just four days after surgery. My beautiful daughter spent the day caring for me, as I had cared for her for so many years. It is a blessing indescribable to begin emerging on the other side of despair, especially when for so long, I was certain I could not.

Exodus 17

Amalek came and fought with Israel at Rephidim. So Moses said to Joshua, "Choose for us men, and go out and fight with Amalek. Tomorrow I will stand on the top of the hill with the staff of God in my hand." So Joshua did as Moses told him, and fought with Amalek, while Moses, Aaron, and Hur went up to the top of the hill. Whenever Moses held up his hand, Israel prevailed, and whenever he lowered his hand, Amalek prevailed. But Moses' hands grew weary, so they took a stone and put it under him, and he sat on it, while Aaron and Hur held up his hands, one on one side, and the other on the other side. So his hands were steady until the going down of the sun. And Joshua overwhelmed Amalek and his people with the sword.

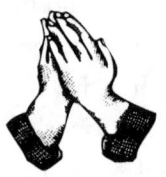

Breathing the Scent of Distant Memories

July 27, 2016

I spent part of the day going through files and storage cabinets in preparation to sell our house. We are downsizing to a riverside condo if all goes as planned. I won't tell you about pouring through decades of artwork, awards, writing projects, homemade cards, and diaries from my kids and twenty-five years of homeschooling. I won't dwell on the buckets of tears and heaving sobs as I remembered how much I loved my children and tried so *so* hard to be a perfect mom to them, as well as a perfect teacher through all twelve years of schooling each one of them.

Instead, I will tell you about artwork from the 90's that I had totally forgotten I had done! I found them in a sketchbook. Back then, I had a small travel watercolor set, and everywhere I went, I painted a watercolor!

Frankly, I was flabbergasted. I had two young sons by then. How had I been able to take them to all these beautiful places, paint the scenery, and somehow keep those boys alive and content?

I don't remember. Maybe they *weren't* content. I do remember the places. The watercolor paintings brought back vivid emotions I felt at the time in the midst of such beauty.

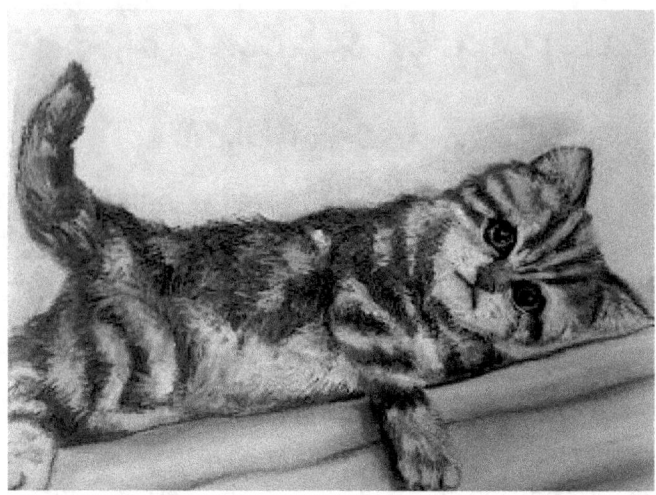

And who is this cat? Is it my little tiger kitten Denali? It might be. I don't remember doing this pastel but it is clearly my work. It's strange looking back at a lifetime of painting. I never thought I was very good...I just knew I HAD to produce art. But looking back, I was not bad.

Some of the names on the paintings were of places I didn't remember. Villagio? Auburn Park? Shove Park? Yet my boys were in many of the paintings so we must have gone to those places and played, as the paintings depicted...like my oldest son digging in the sand of a park beach I could not conjure back from the ghostly images in my head of a faded past.

Many paintings were of places embedded clearly in my mind, like my parents' lake house I loved so well. I captured little details, like wildflowers along the shoreline, or my second boy, Matthias, hooking a worm on his fishing pole. Such good, wonderful memories!

And then I came across some old photos of me and my beloved Honeybun, and of hubby and me. All of us looked sprite, and young, and carefree. Had we really ever felt that way?

After hours of weeping and weeding through memories, I went to my radiology appointment. They marked my chest for the exact area the radiation beam would be directed to zap out any potential lingering breast cancer. I lay still in the CAT scan, eyes closed, thinking of my paintings of all the beautiful places we'd visited, my young children, and the dreams of youth. The machine whirred and clunked noisily, but I breathed deeply the distant scent of hope and optimism and remembered I had done my best. It wasn't perfect, but it was my best. I hope that is what they remember when I am gone.

Joel 2:25

I will restore to you the years that the swarming locust has eaten, the hopper, the destroyer, and the cutter, my great army, which I sent among you.

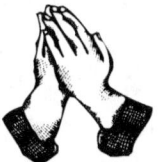

Hiding Behind God

July 29, 2016

Yesterday, the daughter of a mom I work with who chose life over abortion was born mid-morning. I received her picture in a text message right before my doctor appointment. The mama is ecstatic but exhausted. I felt the usual overwhelming joy that this little girl might have never seen her birthday if it wasn't for us sidewalk counselors at the busy abortion center. A second mama I had counseled also went into labor. Many people have been involved in this young lady's amazing decision to choose life, so we were all anxiously in prayer. The onslaught of new life was good fortification as I headed in to see my oncology plastic surgeon.

I was seeing him the first time in a month since he did phase two of my breast reconstruction. He was pleased. My blood pressure was back to its healthy low normal. My scars look great. All is well in how the new breast is healing. I no longer have to wear my compression shorts (though he felt they were quite stylish as far as compression shorts go...). I am cleared to bike ride.

That's where the good news ended.

NO kayaking for a month. No sitting in or cooling off in the lake till after radiation is completed. Radiation begins August 8 and lasts six full weeks, every day except weekends. There is NOTHING I can do to determine whether I get severe scarring from the radiation or not. It is 'luck'. Some women scar a lot, some just a little. *All* will scar (internal breast scarring called capsular contraction). If it is painful or extensive, I need to START ALL OVER with a muscle flap from my back to reconstruct the breast.

All I can do is pray. And ask you all to pray for me if you think of it...

Oh, and one last tidbit, sometimes women go three years without problems, and *then* scars form, and they need another surgery.

I blinked at the doctor. At least he doesn't try to sugarcoat anything. I appreciate his honesty. He told me before the last surgery that the liposuction to my thighs to harvest fat for my breast would leave me feeling like I had been hit by a truck. I thought he was kidding. He wasn't.

He was right. The only thing I would have added to his prediction of how I would feel post-liposuction is this: *you will feel like you have been hit by a LARGE truck with SHARP spikes all over the fender.*

Now one month post-surgery, my thighs only hurt *a little*. They DO still hurt. Nothing like how much they hurt for the first two weeks, but...wow. If you are thinking of this as an option to trimming your figure for vanity purposes --*just say no to liposuction.*

Back to radiation. I am really hoping to defy the odds and be one of the few with zero to minimal scarring from the radiation treatment.

Meanwhile, I reread my blog from yesterday about how BIG God is. He is BIG....REALLY BIG. Bigger than a large truck, bigger than cancer, bigger than radiation scars. He is so big, that if you need a refuge, God is the place to run. I intend to be hiding behind Him.

<u>Psalm 62:8</u>

Trust in him at all times, O people; pour out your heart before him; God is a refuge for us.

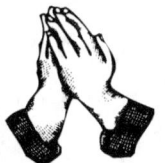

How Cleaning a Closet Helped Me During a Melt Down

August 4, 2016

I cannot believe how fast the publisher got the print book of my brand new book to me. It came at a perfect time. While in general, I am upbeat and hopeful on the breast cancer journey, I start radiation August 8, and I was having a minor melt-down day. This happens now and then, when what I am facing overwhelms me. God sent me a message to lead me through this stormy day. It involved cleaning my closet.

If you saw my newly culled and cleaned closet, I am sure you could not tell I had worked all day to clean it. It is still pretty stuffed.

However, some areas are miraculously clean. The upper shelves were stuffed to the ceiling with clothes and odds and ends, but now are completely empty. I really thought I would NEVER get through it all, but I did.

There were many lessons in downsizing to move into a home half the size of our current home. Cutting in half the impossible accumulation of things is not a task anyone *wants* to tackle, let alone someone just five weeks out of her second major surgery for breast cancer, with lifting and stress restrictions. However, I discovered the key to doing any terrible, overwhelming task.

Just get started.

I am serious. If you are like 99.9% of the people on earth, you have a whole bundle of things you are avoiding. You procrastinate and find other ways to fill your time and sidestep the task because you cannot imagine tackling such an impossible ordeal. I know. That is how I have felt for years as I walked by my closet. It is how I felt facing cancer, raising children, house-training the dog...sometimes even rolling out of bed to face a particularly difficult day. All of us have those *bury our face in the sand* moments because the picture on our screen is chock full of angst. Easier to turn it off.

So. The closet. Everything that didn't have a good place to be stored went in my closet. Yet, if we are ever really going to downsize and follow the dream of a waterfront home where I can kayak right off my doorstep, I had to stop avoiding the closet.

Is there Biblical advice on *doing* instead of *avoiding*? LOTS.

Here are a smattering:

What good is it, my brothers, if someone says he has faith but does not have works? Can that faith save him? If a brother or sister is poorly clothed and lacking in daily food, and one of you says to them, "Go in peace, be warmed and filled," without giving them the things needed for the body, what good is that? So also faith by itself, if it does not have works, is dead. James 2:14-17

For if anyone is a hearer of the word and not a doer, he is like a man who looks intently at his natural face in a mirror. For he looks at himself and goes away and at once forgets what he was like. But the one who looks into the perfect law, the law of liberty, and perseveres, being no hearer who forgets but a doer who acts, he will be blessed in his doing. James 1: 23-25

But someone will say, "You have faith and I have works." Show me your faith apart from your works, and I will show you my faith by my works. James 2:18

Little children, let us not love in word or talk but in deed and in truth. 1 John 3:18

Now in general, these verses are talking about faith being put in action. I don't think it is a huge leap to generalize this to action tackling hard things in the way I am suggesting. If something must be done, you cannot pray it away. No matter how much faith you have, if you are *able* to do what is required, you should do it.

I have an excellent example. I have spoken to countless people who tell me how important the work is that Cities4Life volunteers do on the sidewalks of the abortion mill.

"But *I* could never do it," they tell me, "I will pray for you."

"There are many things you could do to help if you feel you can't be on the sidewalk. You could be a mentor to the mamas, send them Bible verses, help organize the baby showers, help galvanize churches to walk alongside these mamas, help us find food and clothing resources, donate to the organizations actively helping these moms make a decision for life..."

"I will pray about it."

Then I never hear from them again.

Now don't get me wrong. Prayer is pivotal in our relationship with God, but I can't help but feel sometimes we are hiding behind prayer. Action is too scary, and too messy. Easier to sit back and pray...and hope someone else will do what needs doing.

So. Back to my closet.

I took a deep breath, and launched. I emptied the entire top shelf of one side of the closet. Piece by piece, I separated the items into *save, garbage, and donate.* It took a long time. I am the queen of forcing things into every nook and cranny so words can not give a full picture of the hopeless state of my overfilled closet.

For three full days, this was my strategy. Take one section at a time and separate the contents into the three piles. As soon as that section was complete, throw out the garbage pile, bring the donation pile to Goodwill, and neatly return the save pile, or store in clearly marked bins. If I didn't do it immediately, my save pile mysteriously returned to full size again. At first, I was certain I would spend the rest of my life cleaning my closet.

Gradually, the joy of a neat, orderly, organized little room began to grip me and what had been impossible became achievable.

On top of that, emptying my closet led to so much unexpected joy. Look at some of the things I found:

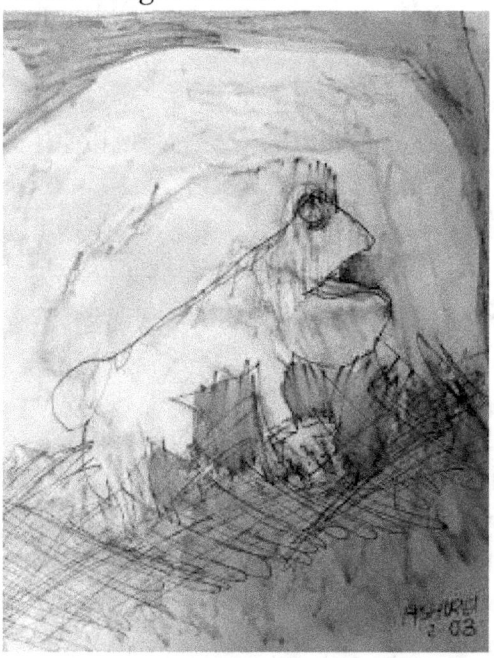

Asherel was five when she painted this frog. I found tons of her artwork from her youngest years through young teens.

I had so much fun looking at her old school work, art, and her diaries. She was five when she wrote a hilarious essay about a duck-dog. If I hadn't cleaned my closet, I wouldn't have found it. I wouldn't have laughed and remembered parts of life that I had long ago forgotten.

When I had all the dust and memories I could stand, I loaded my bicycle in my van. I drove out to the lake shore where one day I hope to live. I wanted to see if we really *did* move to the tiny lake condo, would I enjoy biking in that area?

Yes. It was heaven. All this cleaning and purging of possessions will be worth it. I'm glad I forced myself to get started. You should stop avoiding whatever it is you have to do and just don't know how to begin. BEGIN. Honestly, you will feel better in the long run.

And don't think I don't want prayer for the six full weeks of radiation I am about to endure. Please pray. This is one of the areas where prayer is totally called for!

<u>Proverbs 14: 23</u>

All hard work brings a profit, but mere talk leads only to poverty.

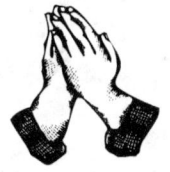

What Conquers Fear

August 8, 2016

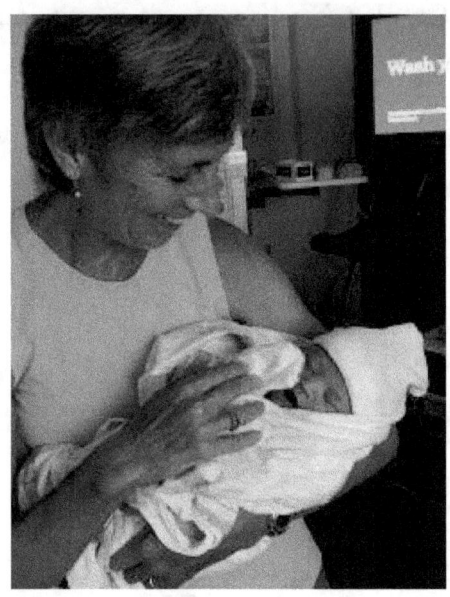

Yep. Doesn't get much better than this.

Below is the text I got yesterday, from a mama and daddy that I have counseled extensively since they chose life over abortion through our presence on the sidewalks of the abortion center. When the text arrived, I was stressing a little about my radiation treatments for breast cancer which start (gulp) today:

Mama: *A healthy boy, 7.8 pounds, and 21 inches!*

Me: *Oh he is gorgeous! Thank you so much for letting me know and sending me the pictures of your beautiful baby.*

Mama: *Of course. I had to let u know! U are part of the reason y he's here with us today....thanks a million- we love u Ms.Vicky.*

Me: *Love you too!!! Stay in touch!*

Mama: *We sure will. They will be discharging tomorrow-- if u would like to come by and visit him, u are more than welcome to.*

No one had to ask me twice! It was an hour drive to the hospital, but nap forgotten, I was in the car within five minutes. Holding a newborn baby sure beat obsessing about the woes of radiation. Even if the little baby was struggling with gas and cried most of the visit. I'd take a crying baby over radiation any day.

After the visit:

Me: *It was such a joy to see you all. Thank you for inviting me. It really meant a lot.*

Mama: *U r welcome ...u are special to us*

Me: *The feeling is mutual! Hugs and prayers to both of you.*

I had been in a funk. I don't like to admit this. I want to be inspiring. It is not inspiring to be overwhelmed with fear, sorrow, and worry. I do not want to undergo radiation. I am so afraid of what this potent treatment will do to my lungs, the newly healed breast, scars, implant, my energy level, and my skin. I have been quite emotional for days, trying to pray and walk the fear away through ten-mile-walks on my beloved Greenway. I slept little Saturday night, filled with angst.

I was just drifting off to sleep, sort of watching the Olympics, when I got the text about the new little baby. This mama is very dear to me. She is so vulnerable and sweet, and is trying very hard to walk with the Lord. She has needed extensive help from Cities4Life and they have provided it. The young couple and the baby might not have made it without our intervention.

I cannot take credit for it. God gets ALL the glory...but I am ecstatic to be used by Him on this mission. As I drove to the hospital, held the baby, and drove home, I never once thought about how grieved I was over the prospect of radiation. All I thought about was how incredibly grateful I was that this new little life was here on Earth, and I had played a part in it through God's gracious divine appointment.

John 12:26

If anyone serves me, he must follow me; and where I am, there will my servant be also. If anyone serves me, the Father will honor him.

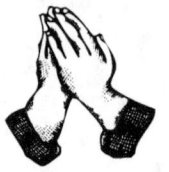

A Tale of Two Choices

August 9, 2016

I was very nervous yesterday about my upcoming radiation session. It was just a dry run, with x-rays marking the area to be radiated, and educating me on the daily process as well as handling side effects. It was a long session, but the actual radiation doesn't start till today. I was already upset when I went in, partly from fear of this new unknown but also because of financial concerns the cancer has brought us. So when I settled in the little room with the nurse, I started crying almost immediately.

She was *beyond* kind and quickly picked up that I was a Christian. She shared with me that she too was a believer and her deep faith was helping her through some very difficult issues, similar to my own. She has come through to the other side of that trial and emerged victorious. She understood my fears and my tears, and spoke about her own grief and crying over her situation. She assured me, this was not from lack of faith, but from the overflow of the emotions devastating news brings. She rejoiced knowing that God had sent me to her, a divine appointment, knowing she had a message that would be what I needed to hear.

"I am here to tell you you will do fine, just like I did."

I began crying again, not out of fear anymore but out of gratitude to God for sending me someone who so beautifully understood what I was going through and could provide the comfort that was exactly what I needed at exactly the right time.

Before the doctor appointment, I had gone to the abortion center sidewalks to speak on behalf of the babies, knowing I could not stay long because of my radiation appointment. The demons were really riled! Two women became incredibly angry with me while I was speaking on the microphone and charged me, one throwing her purse to the ground on her way to pummel me. She was livid, vile, and said that she wanted to go to hell because it was so much more fun than the world we lived in following God. I was not afraid, though I was pretty sure I was about to be attacked. Fortunately, her friend grabbed her, talked her down, and she retreated.

I do not mind when people get angry with me for speaking the truth I feel God has called me to speak. I would much rather have them become angry than be indifferent. I think their anger means there's a conscience that is pricked, and that they can still be reached.

Two moms that we know of chose life for their babies. I would have liked to have seen the outcome of what happened with the angry young woman, but I had to go to my doctor appointment.

Originally, my radiologist had told me I would need 33 radiation treatments, but that was downgraded to 30, so I will be done with radiation September 20. There will be much rejoicing on that day, but there was even rejoicing at that first session yesterday, seeing how God planted Comfort and Hope in my path.

I remembered the nurse's advice as I lay for twenty minutes on the radiation table. They x-rayed me, then a grid of green lines was beamed onto my chest and they drew all over me with purple markers. (That is the area I am to apply a special cream to help with the inevitable skin irritation.) As I lay there while machines moved all around me taking photos and doing who-knows-what, I thought of what the nurse said: "During my treatments, I would imagine that the radiation beam was God's warmth, God's healing hand upon me, and I would thank Him for my healing."

The woman who was so angry at the abortion center justified her decision to abort based on bad circumstances in her life, including domestic violence. I find it ironic that she wanted to go to hell where it was "more fun". I imagine hell is peopled with those unrepentant, hard, rebellious, God-defying hearts that have caused her so much pain in this life on earth.

The contrast between that woman and my nurse was quite striking.

The first woman: vile words and foaming anger, cursing God for her struggles, and desiring to go to hell rather than do what she knew God was calling her to do. Circumstances define her *moral choices*.

vs.

My nurse: gentle, compassionate, undergoing a terrible struggle herself but thanking God for it in preparing her to minister to another hurting child of God. Moral, Godly choices define her *circumstances*.

The first woman was a vision of self-inflicted hell, and the other was a vision of Christ-delivered heaven. There is no doubt which side of that stark divide I would rather be on.

"Can I still go on long walks?" I asked the nurse before leaving the session, "I love to walk."

She smiled. "The data shows that the women who have the least side effects are those who exercise."

I lifted my eyebrows. "I often walk ten miles a day. Is that ok?"

"Oh yes, it is encouraged!" she said.

I've got this! With God, and good sneakers, I've got this!

2 Corinthians 1:3-4

Blessed be the God and Father of our Lord Jesus Christ, the Father of mercies and God of all comfort, who comforts us in all our affliction, so that we may be able to comfort those who are in any affliction, with the comfort with which we ourselves are comforted by God.

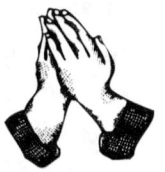

A New Mission Field

August 10, 2016

So, for those of you lucky enough to never need radiation therapy, here is your chance to know what it is like. I was so scared all morning yesterday, prior to my first treatment session. I worked on a pastel painting to keep my mind off the torture I was certain I would have to endure. I also started the sequel to my latest new novel. I am so grateful I have a creative mind that can take me places that are so much more pleasant than my reality.

I was petrified as I changed into my gown and sat down to await my fate. I was certain the machine would malfunction and I would be burned to a crisp. They came to get me and I notified them immediately that I was very scared. They assured me there was nothing to be afraid of.

"Fine...then let's trade places, shall we?" Surprise, surprise, no takers on my offer.

They positioned me on the bed of torture and offered a washcloth to put over my eyes.

"No thanks, I am fine."

Stupid, stupid, stupid. Always take whatever comfort is offered.

The lights that come on last a long time and you can see them through your (clenched tightly shut) eyelids. Sometimes they are bright blood red and seep into all the cracks in your brain. Sometimes they are neon green and feel like a drug flashback. Sometimes, they pulse unexpectedly just when you can no longer stand to squeeze your eyes shut a moment longer, and you see they are still there, lurking a little lower, but they find your vulnerable eyeball and blind you.

They told me I would only be on the table *ten minutes tops*, and the treatment itself (a.k.a. dangerous radiation) lasts only a minute or two. I was on the table 45 minutes. NO LIE. I was thinking it was the LONGEST ten minutes I had ever lived through, but I had just prayed that morning that God would not let me wish my life away by wanting terrible things to happen quickly so I could just get them over with.

I got my wish.

It turns out, despite my vague sense throughout that I was being slowly fried like an egg, most of the time was just them waiting through a computer glitch, and then the doctor being on the phone and unavailable. So all those endless minutes while I was envisioning my skin being slowly grilled, *nothing* was going on except the technicians chatting and sipping coffee in the safe room. I suspect they were playing with those excruciatingly bright light switches just to mess with me.

I could have sworn I felt soldering irons burning through my bones. Nope. TOTALLY my imagination. This is the danger of a creative mind. So after enduring forty minutes of sheer terror, thinking I would not live even though it did not hurt at all...they came back in and told me they were now ready to START the treatment.

START???? ARE YOU SERIOUS???

And no offers of washcloths over my eyes this time, which I would have killed my grandmother for, if she were still alive. Which she is not.

When they came back after the treatment, they told me I could now go. I sat up shakily. I told them I felt a tightness in my chest skin. They laughed, politely, and told me I would not feel or see any skin changes for a couple of weeks. The tightness was from holding my arm in the outstretched position for so long, which they apologized for. It would go much smoother and faster from now on.

I returned to the changing room where I met a couple of other women who are old pros at radiation. They were finishing their several weeks of treatment, and assured me, they had had no problems whatsoever. One even showed me her breast, which looked a little red, like a minor sunburn, but that was all.

She was quite social, and soon was telling me about her horses.

"Horses!" I said, "I love horses!! I am an author and I write books about horses!"

She asked for my business card (which I happened to have with me) and I think I made a sale. You never know what benefits might come from radiation.

Fortunately, I had lots of opportunities to share my faith.

"Is there anything I can get you?"

"No, I'll just pray...."

"Would you like to listen to music while you are on the table?"

"Yes, Christian music if you have it."

"Did you have to get chemo?"

"No...it was a miracle. They were certain I would, but praise God, I was spared that."

One of my cancer survivor friends told me radiation would be an opportunity to have a new mission field. She was right. It gave me a sense of purpose in the midst of all that fear.

As I left, I felt like a new woman. I had done it. I had survived my first radiation treatment.

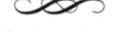

Mark 16:15

And he said to them, "Go into all the world and proclaim the gospel to the whole creation.

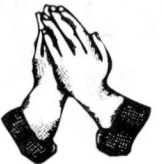

Working the Radiation Room — a Silver Lining

August 11, 2016

Radiation for my second session went much more smoothly than Day One. First of all, I was not scared out of my noggin. Secondly, I accepted the washcloth for my eyes this time so I didn't have to keep them squeezed shut. Thirdly, there was no computer malfunction as on Day One so I was in and out of there within ten minutes.

The sweet technician asked me how my day had gone so far.

"Great! I am an author and I just released my latest novel this morning, I wrote 5,000 words on the new book's sequel."

"Wow!" she said, "What sort of books do you write?"

As I described my books, the second technician came in and was also interested.

Two more potential readers! And I still have five full weeks of radiation to go! I could double my readership by the time I finish with cancer.

Maybe I'll do a book signing outside the chemo room...

Radiation is a quick in-and-out treatment but chemo takes hours. They could use good, clean, inspiring reading material.

While resting under my washcloth, listening to the whir of the radiation machine doing its thing, I was working on my sequel's plot development. I have a very general idea of what will happen, but it is quite vague. I don't know how it will end. Some writers plan it all out with meticulous detail. I usually start writing, and the book develops a life of its own. It rarely goes in ways I expect or plan. It is almost other-worldly, as though someone other than me is in control.

Which is true. Someone other than me *IS* in control. I am really grateful for that. The Holy Spirit indwells me, and guides me, and comforts me. I will blame the Holy Spirit if my new book bombs and doesn't sell. (Just kidding. Any flaws are not the Holy Spirit's but mine...)

Here is the lesson for the day. Who would ever imagine that in a radiation treatment room, God would be at work helping with such a mundane thing as financial security? I am an author. If my books don't sell, I go broke. God knows that. If I must have cancer, the need to make a living doesn't change. How incredibly gracious of God to open doors even in such an unlikely setting.

This is not only true of financial issues, but of *all* issues. If God is really in control, and it would be foolish to presume otherwise, then of course He can work in any environment. Even in a radiation room where so much fear and sorrow resides. That is exactly the sort of quirky place where God reveals His power.

Isaiah 49:3

He said to Me, "You are My Servant, Israel, In Whom I will show My glory."

227

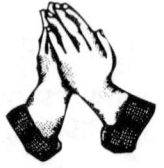

Remorse and Victory

August 13, 2016

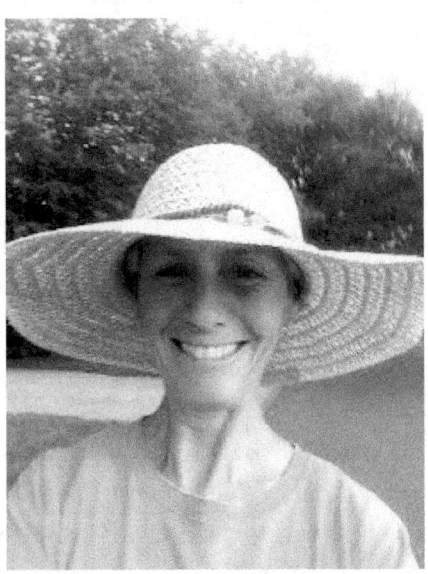

Hubby knew the radiologist wanted me to stay out of the sun for the six weeks of radiation. He also knew I wouldn't. So he got me this super-wide brimmed sunhat for my birthday. I love it. I put it on and went on a walk immediately. It blocks the sun from my face as well as half of the neighborhood.

So no one starts screaming at me, I *am* allowed to be in the sun as long as I block it from the radiated parts of my body. The hat and a high neck t-shirt do that.

I finished my first week of radiation and get the weekend off from melting my skin! Today, I head joyfully to a baby shower for one of the most "high drama" encounters I've ever had at the abortion center where I stand on the sidewalk and encourage mamas to choose life. Due to privacy issues, all I can tell you is it involved coercion by the young lady's family to abort, a police chase, threats to me and my car, driving for an hour trying to find a safe house for the underage mama, and ultimately God working in miraculous ways to save the teen and her baby. Today will be the baby shower that celebrates her tenacity and determination to save her baby no matter the cost.

She doesn't have an easy road ahead of her, but she has shown that she is filled with courage, and she *does* know the Lord. She accepted Jesus as savior when she met us on the sidewalks of the abortion center. Tears poured out of her as she asked Jesus into her life after we shared the Gospel. We prayed with her while demons were rattling the door of our HELP Crisis Pregnancy Center mobile ultrasound RV. Peace reigned within, because as we know from the Bible, "where two or more are gathered in my name, there am I in the midst of them". Jesus blocked all evil influence right on the sidewalk of the Southeast's busiest abortion center.

This sweet mama will win the battle if she keeps Jesus first in her life. I was pondering how deeply I wished *I* had known God from my childhood. I like to think that perhaps I would have made less terrible choices. The sins I committed not only affected me, but had lifelong repercussions to people I didn't even yet know at the time. Sin is a ripple in the water that extends far from the stone that first set it in motion.

We don't really know that when we are young. We have no idea of the extent of damage sin inflicts. I *sure didn't.* Now that I am sixty, I *sure do.*

So on my birthday, I found myself crying buckets of tears, regretful and remorseful for things that happened decades ago that I cannot take back now. All I can do now is feel the sorrow, and ask God for forgiveness. He grants it and removes the stain of sin from the *second* I accept Jesus' sacrifice on the cross. It does not remove my remorse or worldly consequences, but before God, I stand forgiven and redeemed.

As part of my birthday schedule, I instructed my art class of nursing home residents in the use of pastels to render a barn and fields. I showed them that *surprisingly,* it is possible to correct mistakes when using those messy chalk pastels.

"You smudge out the incorrect marks, then spray it with hairspray. After the spray dries, you can go over it with more pastel, and correct the mistake. It is as though you never even made that wrong mark!"

It occurred to me at that moment that I was rehashing my tearful thoughts of my morning walk.

"It is like washing away our sin. When we accept Jesus as Lord, God no longer looks at our sin. It is washed away, and He sees it no more." I hadn't planned to say that...but it poured out of me.

A few residents nodded. One smiled. No one grew upset. Old people know how much we all long to wash away the sins of our impetuous youth.

Isaiah 1:18

"Come now, let us reason together, says the Lord: though your sins are like scarlet, they shall be as white as snow; though they are red like crimson, they shall become like wool.

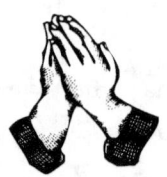

Ashes to Beauty

August 14, 2016

Joy on several fronts yesterday. First, I kayaked for the first time in seven weeks since my cancer surgery. I cried when I pulled up to my kayaking launch site. It felt like I was seeing an old friend for the first time in years, a friend I wasn't certain I would ever see again. I paddled very slowly but spent an hour on my beloved lake, communing with herons and singing "When peace like a river attendeth my way..."

When I first pulled up to the lake, and unloaded my kayak, I started sobbing. I hadn't realized that part of me feared I would never kayak again until I pulled my kayak into the lake, and dipped my feet in the warm water. Tears gushed with joy that I was not only *alive*, but about to do one of my favorite activities on earth again.

Secondly, I got to hold a baby that I almost got arrested trying to save. This story is one I cannot tell because the mama is a minor, but after one of the most difficult and drama-filled rescues from abortion I have yet experienced as a sidewalk counselor, this little baby girl nestled in my arms yesterday.

Thirdly, my new book, Unlikely Friends, was the #1 best-seller in horse books on Amazon and the #1 Hot New Release. I checked its rank by accident and could not believe it when I saw the ranking. #1!!! Man that feels good!!! It had sold so slowly upon release that I was very concerned. If my books don't sell, how can I afford to keep writing? I feel certain God has called me to write...but we have a LOT of bills with my cancer diagnosis.

In all three of these events, God took ashes and swirled them into something unexpected, something more beautiful than I could have ever imagined. When we are trudging through deep, grey, suffocating ashes, it is impossible to hope that we will ever breathe clean air again or see a clear sky unsmudged with death, desperation, and decay.

BUT THEN GOD.

Isaiah 61:1-3

The Spirit of the Lord God is upon me, because the Lord has anointed me to bring good news to the poor; he has sent me to bind up the brokenhearted, to proclaim liberty to the captives, and the opening of the prison to those who are bound; to proclaim the year of the Lord's favor, and the day of vengeance of our God; to comfort all who mourn; to grant to those who mourn in Zion— to give them a beautiful headdress instead of ashes, the oil of gladness instead of mourning, the garment of praise instead of a faint spirit; that they may be called oaks of righteousness, the planting of the Lord, that he may be glorified.

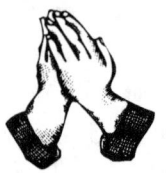

Choose Life! And a million dollar idea might ensue....

August 17, 2016

I had a problem. My radiologist told me I must be sure the area that will be radiated for the next six weeks not be exposed to the sun. I cannot use suntan lotion either or the radiated area will be *REALLY TICKED OFF*. The area extends from just above my clavicle, across and down my chest, and on to portions of my back and underarm. The only thing that covers it fully is a high neck t-shirt.

My problem is I love to kayak and have been given the go-ahead from my surgeon to kayak. However, kayaking in a high neck t-shirt with sleeves is *hot*. I ideally want to wear my bathing suit...but would need some sort of sun protection over the areas that are in the radiation zone which my bathing suit doesn't cover.

I needed a sun cape. A lightweight sun cape that could get wet.

You would think with the huge number of women who have breast cancer that *someone* would have designed such a thing. NO. I looked everywhere. Nowhere on the entire internet is there a sun cape. The closest thing I could find was a cassock for priests...around $350 on sale. And they are not water friendly. Nor cool. (At least not temperature cool. They are the *other* kind of cool, if you ask me.)

I also found costume superhero capes, but they were too long, and not appropriate for water sports. Note: superheroes are Batman, or Spiderman, or Superman...never Fishman. (However, I *did* like the idea of kayaking in a batman cape made for children, impracticable as it was....) Besides, I needed 360 degree coverage. Superhero capes don't usually cover the clavicle and upper chest. I suspect superheroes don't get breast cancer or require radiation therapy.

I contacted my clever daughter who suggested I sew one. "It would be easy," she said. Since it was so easy, I was hoping she would offer to do it, but no offer was forthcoming.

I mused over the problem and had a brainstorm. I took an old t-shirt and cut off the bottom half. Then I cut open the armhole seams. I sewed it so that the open arm seams attached to the sides and *voila*, the t-shirt became a cape! Then I hemmed it with a nice zigzag stitch in contrasting thread. I now had a chic, cost-free sun cape.

However, it was originally a t-shirt with an ugly design I had never liked. It was for a team I had managed years ago, and the design printed on the back was of a skeleton. I didn't want my new sun-cape to have something so depressing as a skeleton on it.

So I found fabric paint from who-knows-when-or-where, and began drawing over and altering the skeleton design. I had thought I would just spend a few minutes, but soon, the design took on a life of its own and I worked for an hour or so.

The result is pictured here.

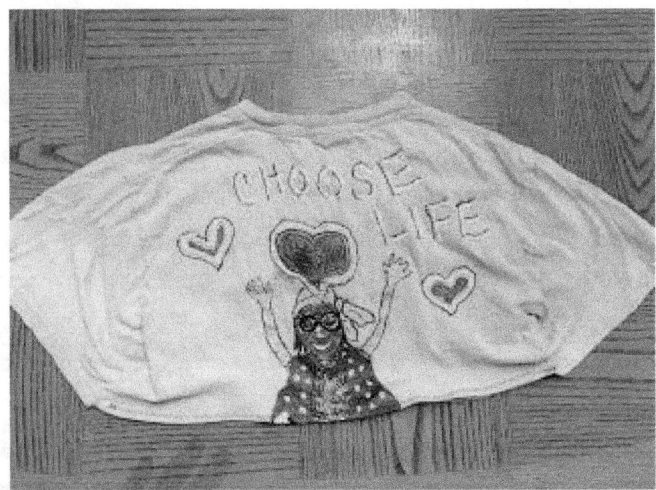

Choose Life.

Choose life when I have cancer, remembering cancer *doesn't have me*. **Choose life** when abortion seems to be the only way out. **Choose life** when God sets before us blessing or curse, life or death. **Choose *eternal life*** in Jesus.

I was so happy. Not only did I have a sun cape that would slip easily over my head, was washable, and made of cool cotton, but the design was creative and unique and said *just* what I wanted to say while kayaking across the peaceful waters of my beloved lake.

I will call it my Son-Cape. I think I may wear it as part of my cities4life uniform when I go each Monday to the abortion center sidewalks to counsel the abortion-minded mamas. I am not a superhero, but I believe my cape is anointed by the One who created those babies and me, and yearns for us to choose life. Choose Him.

Deuteronomy 30:19

I call heaven and earth to witness against you today, that I have set before you life and death, blessing and curse. Therefore choose life, that you and your offspring may live,

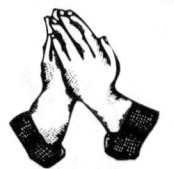

Faith Will Be Sight

August 20, 2016

I finished the second week of radiation! One third of the way through! So far, I feel great but I do notice a slight redness in the radiated area. It is a little early to be seeing skin change, so I hope that is not a bad omen of what is to come.

In the attempt to avoid radiation from the sun, I washed my shirts in a special product that adds SPF protection to clothing. My new invention, the "Son-Cape", went in the special wash load to be sun-proofed as well.

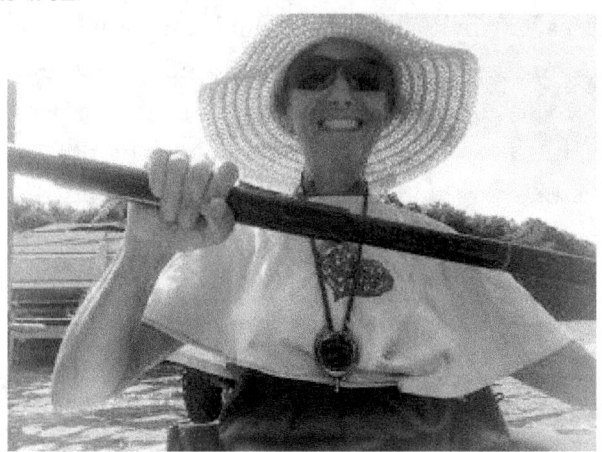

However...how will I know if it really works? There is no visible change to the sun-proofed clothing. I just have to take the manufacturer's word for it. See, *faith* is required in so many areas of life. Faith that the products we buy really will do what they say they do, that the food we eat isn't filled with all kinds of harmful, undetectable chemicals or hormones, that the treatments doctors prescribe don't do more harm inside us than good. I have *faith* that the radiation is killing bad cells and letting good cells live, but I cannot see its invisible work in my body.

Life is one big faith-fest.

The question is not whether we have faith or not...*all* of us have faith. The question is *what* is our faith *IN*? Is it in something worth trusting, and what will be the repercussions if our faith is in the wrong things?

If our faith is in self, or other people, I guarantee we will be disappointed. Others fail us almost as often as we fail ourselves. And all you young, nubile studs and studdesses out there, your lovely body will fail you too. Just wait. If your faith is in good health, good looks, or even your good bank account that stretches into more zeros before the decimal than I will ever see, it will end in disillusionment and despair. Faith in those things will not sustain you in life.

The Bible says that *"faith is the assurance of things hoped for, the conviction of things not seen." Hebrews 11:1*

If this were all the Bible said about faith, we would be misled. I *hope* for many things that are not necessarily in my best interests or in the best interests of others. There are also many things I don't see that I hope for, like a million dollars. True sustaining faith must be more than hoping for unseen things.

The verse in Hebrews continues on:

For by it the people of old received their commendation. By faith we understand that the universe was created by the word of God, so that what is seen was not made out of things that are visible.

This clarifies matters a bit. It is by faith we are commended by God. Our faith is not in trivial matters but in the very one who created the entire universe. Furthermore, it is by this faith that we understand the *source* of all things. A very important point is made here. The universe was created out of unseen things and became seen.

There will be a day when our faith will be rewarded. All will be revealed unequivocally. For those who put their faith in Jesus, they will see Him face to face, for all eternity. Those who chose to put their faith elsewhere will be more than disappointed!

Even more importantly, what is the *outcome* of faith in the right thing?

Here is a key verse:

The outcome of your faith, the salvation of your souls. 1 Peter 1:9

The only faith worth having does not guarantee earthly health, wealth, or happiness. It guarantees eternity with God, the salvation of our souls. Right now, we don't see it, but we have the assurance of the unseen. One day, what we hope for will be revealed, and we will be so glad we put our faith where it belongs.

It will be as though my Son-Cape suddenly visibly sparkled with sun-protectant angels holding shields that reflected the harmful UV rays. The blind will see. The light will have permanently penetrated the darkness. All will be made whole and perfect as it was intended from the beginning when God's first reported words to creation were: Let there be light.

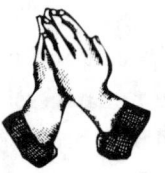

Under God's Grace

August 24, 2016

Yesterday, they finished with the "bolus" in radiation. It had done its job and was being retired. The next month of radiation will not involve the bolus so they asked if I wanted to keep it.

"Why?" I asked.

"Well most women *do* keep them to show their loved ones. No one at home really understands what goes on in radiation, so they bring it home to their husbands or family."

This floored me. I had absolutely NO interest in bringing home my bolus. Let me explain what it is. Maybe I am just weird in not wanting it. The bolus is a plastic piece that fits over the reconstructed breast. They radiate with the bolus in place, and then they take it off and radiate some more. I have no idea why, nor do I know why the bolus is only used the first two weeks.

I *do* know that they all commented on how perfectly the bolus fit. They seemed surprised by this, since every time a new technician put the bolus on me, they remarked on the perfect fit.

Perhaps that is why they seemed surprised when I told them, "No thank you."

What does one *do* with a bolus, even if one is *not* downsizing in preparation of cutting their living space in half? Use it for a Halloween costume? A wall decoration? A pot holder? A soup bowl? I just could not envision any good reason to keep my bolus, though I felt bad that this seemed to upset the radiologist technician who I really like. Maybe not all boluses fit as perfectly as mine.

So far, radiation is having no ill effects on me. There is a slight "sunburn" on the radiated area, but otherwise, I feel nothing out of the ordinary. While it disrupts my afternoon, it is mostly thus far a non-issue. In fact, I was working on an illustration job and totally lost track of time. I almost missed my radiation session because I was transported to the 18th century by my drawing. It was a rude awakening to glance at my watch and realize I was in the 21st century and about to be late for my high tech cancer treatment.

Unfortunately, from this point forward symptoms are supposed to get worse. Skin issues and fatigue are the most likely concerns. I may be one of the lucky ones that get by with nothing more severe than the mild sunburn I already have. That is my prayer.

I lay in bed last night and thanked God for how gently He has treated me through this whole ordeal. It could have been so much worse, and *is* much worse for many women. I don't take enough time to thank God for His gentleness with me. What I deserve is Hell, and what I get is Grace. This is true of all of us.

The older I get, the more I regard sin with horror. I cannot believe how blind I was to the terrible effects of selfishness, pride, arrogance, envy, anger...to name a few of my failings. I still fall prey to all of them, but am usually quicker to despair and repent. Before I became a Christ-follower, I never gave those traits a moment's thought.

No, I don't deserve Grace...but I am grateful.

2 Corinthians 12:9

But he said to me, "My grace is sufficient for you, for my power is made perfect in weakness." Therefore I will boast all the more gladly of my weaknesses, so that the power of Christ may rest upon me.

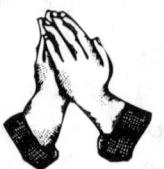

Realigning Perspective

August 25, 2016

It is very easy to become caught up in the *poor, pitiful me* syndrome, and think your world is the worst place on earth. I have been there. We all have, where we know others *may possibly somehow* have a worse time than we do, but it doesn't matter. *Our* worst time belongs to *US,* and we are suffering.

I had a small rash from the radiation. No real big deal, but it itched a little. And there was a funny looking spot at the edge of my reconstructed breast that looked like under-skin scar tissue may be forming. I was feeling a little worried and sorry for myself.

I sat down with two other women waiting for radiation. I am getting to slowly know these women since we all have the same designated daily time to show up for radiation. One lady was sparkling, with the inner light that any believer recognizes as being from someone who loves the Lord. We struck up a conversation, and she began sharing what she had been through thus far on her cancer journey.

Unlike me, she had heart complications and heart surgery. Unlike me, she had chemo. Unlike me, she had developed 'cording' - thick scars that limited her range of motion right after her surgery. She showed me pictures of her legs swollen three times their size from chemo, toenails that had fallen off, and a countertop of hair that had come out in huge clumps till she was bald in three days.

"But I'm blessed," she told me, "My doctors were wonderful. I prayed God would send me just the right doctors for me, and He did."

The radiation technician called her away, and another lady sat down. We struck up a conversation. Unlike me, she also had received several months of chemo. Nine out of ten women do fine with the chemo drugs, but not her. She was taken to the ER after the first round of chemo, and discovered the drug had permanently damaged her heart.

"My birthday is this week," she told me, and then she choked up. "Forgive me...I didn't think I would make it to this birthday."

Also unlike me, though she has had as many radiation treatments as I have, she was in excruciating pain. "My skin looks like it's been burned to a crisp. It's black! I can't hardly stand the pain."

Kind of realigns your perspective, doesn't it?

Psalm 118:24

This is the day that the Lord has made; let us rejoice and be glad in it.

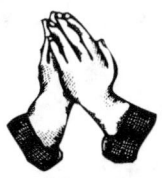

Be Alert, Friends!

August 29, 2016

There is a VERY good reason NOT to fiddle with your phone while riding your bike. Especially a bike with *really* good brakes. Two skinned knees and bruised ribs speak this advice loudly.

I was riding along on my bike with its finely tuned brakes, and was zipping my phone into my bike bag, when I spied a man on my side of the path. Well, okay, it was technically ME who was on HIS side of the path, but why quibble over details?

I braked with one hand. Unfortunately, it was the front wheel brake, and it was *very* responsive. It slammed the front of my bike to a stop, hurling me onto the handlebars and then the pavement. I haven't crashed on my bike in 35 years, and it could have been MUCH worse. My knees were bruised and skinned, but my hands and head escaped unscathed. My rib just under the mastectomied breast took a pounding, and it hurt quite a bit. I don't think I broke it...but I sure bruised it.

I called my radiation nurse.

"Kitty, I did something really stupid and am wondering if I am able to radiate a badly bruised rib?"

She told me to come in early and the doc would assess. She also urged me to be gentle on myself. I guess she saw no good purpose in berating myself for foolishness.

But it *was* foolish and I learned a lesson. Keep my hands on the wheel (handlebars) and my attention on the task at hand. No texting while biking. No doing anything while biking except enjoying the scenery and being alert.

No more selfies on my bike unless I am standing still, no matter how well they make important adjunct illustrations to my blog. Stay focused and keep the main event the main event.

I am lucky I didn't blow out my new breast implant. The poor breast has had enough problems with cancer and two operations. It sure didn't need a bruising bike crash as well. If I had smashed into the handlebar a mere one inch higher, I am pretty sure the new breast would have exploded. The doc agreed.

God was warning me, as I have gotten lax about fiddling with my phone while biking. What can happen? I am only two feet from the ground on a bike, and I never go fast. Well, I saw what could happen. I was spared the most dire consequences, but it could have been very terrible.

The Bible is full of warnings to be alert to the enemy. We are not to let our guard down, and we are to be prepared always. Jesus will return at any time, and He should find us doing what we should be doing, with expectant and purposeful living. We should not be distracted by the things of this world. We should be watchful. He could return at any moment and we should think about what He will find us doing...or not doing.

In other words, pay attention! Focus on doing the right thing, always prepared for whatever may come your way. Be actively seeking righteousness, and flee from evil.

The nurse looked over my injury. Since there was little visible bruising, she told me I could do radiation as scheduled and told me to take Aleve all weekend to reduce swelling and pain. I took a pill right after my appointment, and it worked instantly. I was tempted to text everyone while driving. We all know how stupid that would be.

Stay alert, friends! Jesus is coming soon.

<u>Ephesians 6:18</u>

Praying at all times in the Spirit, with all prayer and supplication. To that end keep alert with all perseverance, making supplication for all the saints,

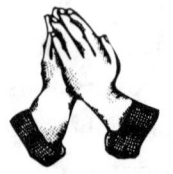

Beautiful Hope

August 30, 2016

Shortly after I arrived on the sidewalks of the busy abortion center where we encourage women to choose life, I spied a little baby lizard running in circles in the middle of the road. I tried to shoo him across the road so he wouldn't be killed by the speeding cars of abortion–minded mamas. He jumped onto my shoe and began to climb up my leg. I took this as an omen or message from God. So I scooped him up instantly, took his photograph, and carried him safely to the other side of the road, away from that terrible evil place.

"They are God's creatures too," I said to my sidewalk cohort, Sherry.

Out of the ground the Lord God formed every animal of the field and every bird of the air, and brought them to the man. The man gave names to all. Genesis 2:19,20

Are not five sparrows sold for two pennies? Yet not one of them is forgotten in God's sight. Luke 12:6

After my volunteer work, I went for my radiation session where I complained to everyone who would listen about the pain in my rib. (The rib is a casualty of a close encounter with my bicycle handlebar. The radiation is from a close encounter with cancer.)

After the doctor examined me, he agreed it was probably broken. There's nothing they can do but if it doesn't improve pain-wise in the next few days they will switch around how they do the radiation to give it a chance to heal. He told me if it is not feeling better, they will need to take a closer look to see if there's maybe something else going on.

"Like what?" I asked

"Oh scarring, fat tissue necrosis."

Lovely.

I thought of the verse about God remembering even the sparrows.

As I closed my eyes during radiation, I envisioned the baby lizard scooped up by a giant hand and carried to safety. A beautiful picture filled my heart of how God performs the same supernatural rescue of me.

He lifted me out of the slimy pit, out of the mud and mire; he set my feet on a rock and gave me a firm place to stand. Psalm 40:2

All in all, a good day—one human baby was saved and one baby lizard. In the midst of my sidewalk volunteer time, one of the moms I work with who chose life several months ago texted me. She is due in a few weeks. She wanted *me* to choose her baby's middle name! I told her I would be honored and I would think about a special name. The baby's first name is Bella. That means beautiful. So I decided her middle name should be Esperanza which is Spanish for hope. Bella Esperanza. Beautiful hope.

I texted the mama. "How about Bella Esperanza? Beautiful Hope. That is what your baby means to me."

"That is lovely! That will be her name!" the mama said.

That was my message from God for the day.

Proverbs 23:18

Surely there is a future, and your hope will not be cut off.

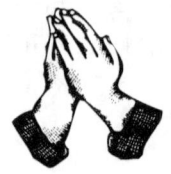

ALL Flesh Shall See the Salvation of God

September 4, 2016

Our old dog Lucky was suffering from bone cancer, and the tumor finally became so large and painful that we had to help usher him to Heaven yesterday. It was a terribly difficult decision, but the vet was clear that it was time. He follows on the paws of our other dog, Honeybun, who died just six months ago, also from cancer. Cancer has been a real spoil sport in our home this year.

Honeybun was too burdened by a traumatic past, and Lucky was too neurotic and socially incompetent for them to have ever quite hit it off. I envisioned them being best friends, and playing together all day. That never happened, though they came to an understanding. They usually slept near each other, and Honeybun tolerated Lucky's incessant fawning over her and licking her broken ear until she would emit a low growl. Then he would back off....temporarily.

Both dogs taught me many things, and both had their individual challenges. Lucky was a consummate escape artist. We spent the first twelve years of his life finding new and increasingly ugly ways of barricading him in the huge backyard which was never huge enough for him. He dug, climbed, jumped, or squeezed his way out nearly every day. Neighbors all knew Lucky because they were forever returning him to our house.

Meanwhile, Honeybun had a quick trigger to aggression, probably based on her need to scrape out a living in the wild where we suspect she had been dumped the year or so before we found her. Lucky, clueless to her cues to leave her alone, constantly sought her attention, licking her, or nudging her, or sniffing her. She attempted to kill Lucky several times, until our hard work with a gifted trainer finally bore fruit. (That often hilarious, and harrowing struggle began my writing career with my best-selling first book I'm Listening with A Broken Ear.)

I had to abandon my dreams of them playing together in lieu of just praying they let each other live.

I envision them now restored to what God intended them to be all along. Honeybun no longer has a broken ear or a troubled past that causes aggressive behavior. Lucky no longer feels the need for incessant attention...nor does he want to escape any more. As my sister mentioned, he has pulled off the final escape, and where else would he want to go? Maybe Heaven was what he was searching for all along. I see them tumbling and running unimpeded together, perfect and whole...like all of us will be if we put our faith in Jesus and enter eternity with Him.

I will see my beloved dogs again. The Bible is filled with references to animals in Heaven. All dogs go to Heaven. If the promise of eternity with Jesus isn't compelling enough, the fact that our dear dogs will be waiting with wagging tails seals the deal for me.

Meanwhile, on my own cancer front, I have finished four weeks of radiation. Week one was uneventful except for the overwhelming fear that I would be melted alive. Week two I got 'folliculitis' which is irritation of hair follicles in the chest/underarm area. Think: itchy hives. Week three I crashed my bike for the first time in thirty-five years and broke my rib just under the reconstructed breast. (Yes. It hurt as much as you are imagining.) Week four my dog died. I am anticipating my last two weeks of radiation with fear and joy, knowing God (and my dogs) are in Heaven cheering me onward.

Job 12:7-10

"But ask the animals, and they will teach you, or the birds of the air, and they will tell you; or speak to the earth, and it will teach you, or let the fish of the sea inform you. Which of all these does not know that the hand of the LORD has done this? In his hand is the life of every creature and the breath of all mankind."

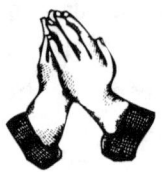

Beautiful Promises of God

September 6, 2016

I napped two hours yesterday. I *only* nap when I am sick. All you 'type A' personalities understand. But I'm not sick. However, I was warned that radiation can cause fatigue. Especially in the last two weeks. I am entering the last two weeks of my six weeks of radiation therapy. I am not so tired that I cannot function, but clearly, there is some fatigue.

Now, it could be I am tired of being in pain with every deep breath I take from my broken rib. Or it could be that I am worried about all the moms who chose life over abortion that I work with. Two of them are in crisis, and there is little I can do but pray. I have been exploring options on how to help them and it is not easy.

Fortunately, there are also moms I work with that are doing well. One of them asked me if I could be with her when her baby is born. I told her if I was in town, I would be thrilled to be there for her. I have never seen a live birth. I didn't really see my three kids get born. I was *there*, of course, but so involved in the mechanics of bringing them safely into the world that I didn't *observe* any of it. It will be exciting to be on the other side of the birth experience. Less painful too.

That same mom told me she has been sharing on Facebook how she almost aborted. She said it made her feel a little ashamed at first, but then, she realized that she was influencing others to make a life-affirming choice. She knew this was one of the missions she and her baby were being called upon to do for God.

She's also the one who asked me to come up with a middle name for her child. She loved the name I initially suggested, but a family member had been hurt by someone with that name, so the mom asked if I could come up with another.

I thought of what the baby means to the mom. The mama wants her baby's first name to be Bella...which means *beautiful*. I suggested *Gracia,* Spanish for 'grace', as the middle name though my heart really wanted *Promessa.* That is Spanish for Promise, so the name would mean 'beautiful promise.' That is what the baby represents in my eyes -- the beautiful promises of God of redemption and eternal life when we follow Him. However, I figured *Promessa* was probably too strange.

The mama didn't like 'Gracia'. She had actually already considered it and rejected it.

"Well, I have one other idea," I said, "What about *Promessa?* I know it is a little unusual..."

"Beautiful promise! *I love it!!!!*" the mama said, "Bella Promessa! Yes!"

She understood instantly why it was such a perfect name for her baby.

Re-energized, I headed out for a walk, thinking of all the beautiful promises of God.

2 Peter 1:4

By which he has granted to us his precious and very great promises, so that through them you may become partakers of the divine nature, having escaped from the corruption that is in the world because of sinful desire.

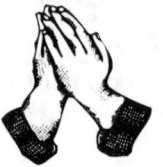

Fashionista of the Senior Set

September 7, 2017

I have arrived. *Fashionista of the Senior Set.* I walked to Walgreens in my homemade Son-Cape, as I have noticed that it is cooler to wear that over a sleeveless shirt rather than wear a high-necked short sleeve t-shirt. I must keep my radiation zone protected from the sun, or the skin reacts angrily. My understanding is that cancer survivors undergoing radiation must continue to keep the radiated skin protected from the sun for *years* following treatment, or the skin can react as though it were being scorched from radiation again. My Son-Cape blocks the ultraviolet rays of the sun, and allows me to wear cooler sleeveless shirts.

I suspect I will be making a few more of my clever Son-Capes over the next few years.

Anyway, back to Walgreens. I was checking out when a teen worker walked by.

"OH wow!" she said, looking at me, "That is such a cool thing to do with a t-shirt! I *love* it! It is adorable."

I was wearing a lime-green belly pack to match my Son-Cape. (As my sweet daughter-in-law told me recently, "I hear belly packs are coming back in style.") This belly pack is particularly useful as it also has a water bottle carrier on it.

The complimentary teen was *not* a dork, either. She had a pierced nose and a few earrings. This was a trendy teen and I had been approved. *Do not be surprised* to see t-shirts converted to Son-Capes on the Paris haute-couture runways this fall. I suspect I won't be given credit, but Givenchy and Christian Dior know the truth.

I went on from my fashion conquest to begin my fourth week of radiation treatment. The technician told me just four more days of the full area radiated and then five days of "boost" to just the breast itself. This is very good news. The doctor told me the worst is over, and I have sailed through radiation treatment with my skin looking really good, and barely any fatigue - the top two side effects with radiation.

"If you hadn't broken your rib, this would be a breeze," he told me. To my relief, according to Dr. Bobo, I should not expect any worse skin reactions or fatigue. It looks like I will survive radiation!

And he is right. Radiation would have been *fine* if it weren't for my broken rib. My rib hurt so badly yesterday morning that I had to go back on the pain meds. However, as long as I take one Aleve in the morning, I am fairly comfortable all day. It could be worse. I must remind myself of that often. However, doc says if it gets worse, he really ought to x-ray to be sure nothing else is going on. I hate to add x-ray radiation to my daily radiation, but when the pain meds wore off this morning, it REALLY hurt.

Let's go on to happier thoughts. After yesterday's radiation treatment, I went on a bike ride, careful to avoid any activity on my bike that might break any more ribs.

Yes, I took a selfie on my bike, but it is not dangerous to do so. My phone is mounted on a secure mount on my handlebar, and there is very little fiddling necessary to take a selfie.

I also finalized plans for my post-radiation celebration. I plan to do an East Coast trip with stops to see both sons, and my parents. I recently discovered the existence of the "Capitol Bike Trail" which begins in Richmond where my son lives. I booked a hotel for two days, so I can spend one full day exploring as much of the 52-mile trail as I can manage. I wrote to the very nice people who oversee the trail, asking about lunch stops and restrooms along the way. Then I told them how thrilled I was to discover their trail, and how I intend to celebrate surviving cancer by biking that trail.

Key to my (mostly) positive outlook since my diagnosis has been finding joy and blessings along the way, as well as setting regular 'rewards', like this bike trip on the Capitol Bike Trail. The blessings have been there throughout this ordeal, but it is easy to lose focus on the good when the bad is SO bad.

Here is my advice: *don't.* Don't lose focus on what is lovely, pure, true, excellent, and worthy. No matter how easy it is to fall into self-pity and despair, *don't.* God is here. You are loved. Eternity awaits your arrival...but maybe not quite yet. Enjoy to the fullest the path to eternity. A joyful heart is good medicine.

And that's why I bought cowboy boots. I ALWAYS wanted cowboy boots. And the salesman told me there was NO REASON why a 60-year-old women should not wear cowboy boots. And picture those beauties WITH my trendy Son-Cape.

Ecclesiastes 5:18

Behold, what I have seen to be good and fitting is to eat and drink and find enjoyment in all the toil with which one toils under the sun the few days of his life that God has given him, for this is his lot.

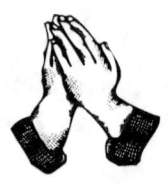

The Upholder of my Life

September 10, 2016

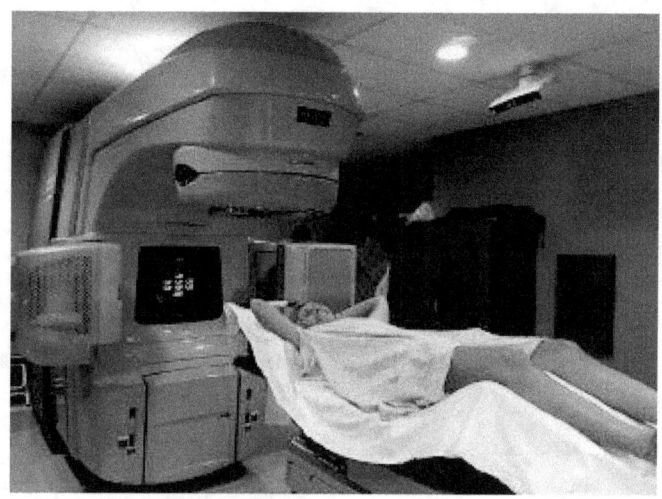

That's me getting ready for my final week of radiation. One more day (Monday) to the already pretty well-cooked area, and then five days to a smaller target area where the actual tumor was, and then I kiss this big, bad machine goodbye. The worst is over. I am not going to blister or shed skin, and the very common side-effect of fatigue has barely grazed me. I am blessed beyond belief.

Furthermore, I have come to almost enjoy the peaceful moments as I am radiated. I lay back in that fairly comfy position, and close my eyes. Since I can be in there for anywhere from five to sometimes twenty minutes depending on whether they need extra photos or *who-knows-what* (not me, and I don't really even *want* to know...), I sometimes enter a dreamy state.

Yesterday, I closed my eyes and as the machine hummed and whined, I suddenly had a revelation. I thought of a GREAT plot direction for my new book. I had been stuck on a slow section, not quite sure how to bring it to life. While radiating, it came to me! I am already a fifth of the way through writing my sequel to Unlikely Friends.

I leaped off the radiation table with a huge smile when the session ended, to the surprise of my radiation technician.

"That was amazing!" I said.

"What?" he asked.

"I know how to write the sticky section of my new book now! It came to me during radiation!"

"Do you think radiation caused it?"

"It must have," I said. "Thank you."

"You're welcome."

If you paid attention, you know how I kicked and screamed about radiation. I was so terrified, and certain all the terrible things that *can* happen, *would* happen. None of them did. Instead, different terrible things happened that were no fault at all of the radiation therapy. Falling off my bike and breaking my rib was in no way related to the cancer or its treatment. It was related to being dumb. I cannot blame that on radiation, much as I would like to.

Anyway, as I went on a walk following radiation, I prayed with deep gratitude to God. I did not want cancer, yet He was with me through all the terrible surgeries. I didn't want complications, yet even the painful and life threatening blood clots did not remove the warmth of His hand in mine. I hardly enjoyed the broken rib right under the newly constructed breast, but even in that, God was present. Impact with my handlebar a centimeter higher, and the whole surgical work might have been destroyed.

What I am saying is I am NOT a strong person. I HATE pain and do not tolerate it well. I could NEVER have endured all I have had to endure without faith in God, and without His very real presence. It has not been EASY, and I sincerely hope I NEVER have to go through any of it again. But...and this is a BIG BUT, *NOTHING IS IMPOSSIBLE WITH GOD.*

Psalm 121:1-8

A Song of Ascents. I lift up my eyes to the hills. From where does my help come? My help comes from the Lord, who made heaven and earth. He will not let your foot be moved; he who keeps you will not slumber. Behold, he who keeps Israel will neither slumber nor sleep. The Lord is your keeper; the Lord is your shade on your right hand. ...

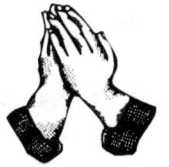

Soul Sickness

September 12, 2016

Great. A *new* malady. It is the final week of radiation. Each week has had an exciting new challenge including radiation fear, radiation rash, folliculitis, broken rib, inner elbow rash, and now for week six: (drum roll please) Golfer's Vasculitis!

This is particularly interesting since I don't golf. Apparently golfing is not required to get Golfer's Vasculitis. I went on a nine-mile walk, and noticed itchy feet about half way through the walk. When I got home and took off my shoes, the tops and soles of my feet had a splotchy, itchy red rash all over them. Here is what an internet site had to say about Golfer's Vasculitis:

The rash is more common in people over 50. Most walkers can't pinpoint anything new they have used that may be causing a reaction. And since so many walkers have it, they couldn't all have contacted the same irritant. The source is simply heat and age--your leg blood vessels getting irritated from the heat.(verywell.com)

Within a couple of hours, the itching was gone, and the rash was still visible, but flattened and less red. More internet research showed that while many radiologists deny it, some radiation patients get rashes outside the radiated area. Perhaps the feet thing *is* Golfer's Vasculitis, or maybe not. I am pretty good at self-diagnosis. However, I do find it curious that at one internet cancer chat site, several cancer patients complained of strange rashes outside the radiation zone. Most said their doctors said it could not have been the radiation causing it. HMMMMM.

I started with a rash in the radiated area, but then got an itchy rash inside my elbows, then the top of my thighs, then my feet, and even a small spot on my neck. The only new thing in my environment is the radiation. I am convinced the radiation has caused all this, as are many radiation patients online who also have experienced these odd rashes.

I am so glad I am almost done with radiation. These seemingly unconnected, mysterious maladies do all point to one thing we *know* to be true. This world is broken. All creation groans with the bondage to decay. We are all covered with the rash of sin and its effects. Many of us look around and wonder what is the cause of all this horror and grief that dogs the world? Like my rash, it keeps popping up in new ways.

Charles Spurgeon described the sickness of sin in his sermon, **A Caution for Sin-Sick Souls** in this way:

Ephraim felt his sickness but he did not know the radical disease that lurked with-in. He saw the local ailment, but was ignorant of the organic derangement of his very vitals. He only perceived the symptoms! He was uneasy, he felt pain, but the discovery did not go deep enough to show him that he was actually dead in trespasses and sins. "He saw his sickness and Judah saw his wound."

Yes, he saw his wound—it smarted and, therefore, his eyes were drawn to the spot. But he did not know how deep it was. He did not know that it had pierced to the heart, that it was, in fact, a death-blow—that the whole head was sick, that the whole heart was faint and that, from the crown of the head even to the sole of the foot, it was all wounds, bruises and putrefying, festering sores! There was but a partial discovery of his lost estate.

The good news: we *will* be set free. There is hope for this ailment that covers us head to foot, but it will not be found on Earth.

In Romans 8, two things are groaning: all creation, and *all of us,* with wordless groans. We are all waiting in anticipation of the redemption of our bodies. We hope, and wait patiently, (uh...ok...), while the Spirit of God helps us, searches our hearts, and then intercedes for us in accordance to God's will. We hope for what we do not yet have, but one day we will. We will be made new, and whole, without blemish or sin, or inexplicable rashes. This makes me think I just might endure the final week of radiation.

Romans 8:18-27

I consider that our present sufferings are not worth comparing with the glory that will be revealed in us. For the creation waits in eager expectation for the children of God to be revealed. For the creation was subjected to frustration, not by its own choice, but by the will of the one who subjected it, in hope that the creation itself will be liberated from its bondage to decay and brought into the freedom and glory of the children of God.

We know that the whole creation has been groaning as in the pains of childbirth right up to the present time. Not only so, but we ourselves, who have the firstfruits of the Spirit, groan inwardly as we wait eagerly for our adoption to sonship, the redemption of our bodies. For in this hope we were saved. But hope that is seen is no hope at all. Who hopes for what they already have? But if we hope for what we do not yet have, we wait for it patiently.

In the same way, the Spirit helps us in our weakness. We do not know what we ought to pray for, but the Spirit himself intercedes for us through wordless groans. And he who searches our hearts knows the mind of the Spirit, because the Spirit intercedes for God's people in accordance with the will of God.

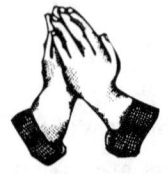

Killing the Old Self

September 14, 2016

Momentous day yesterday. I had the last full radiation session. For the next five days, I have the less invasive targeted radiation, only on the scar itself where apparently the tumors were found. This means the rest of my radiated skin will now begin to heal. It never got very bad. One small square under my arm was quite red, peeling, and hurt a bit, but nothing I couldn't handle. Thus, the worst is over.

My doctor was flummoxed by the strange rashes I have had. He has no idea what they are and why they popped up outside the radiated zone. He told me my theory that my immune system was stressed by radiation, and thus the rashes broke out, was a good thought. He felt that could be the case.

My nurse has never had anyone report strange rashes in the ten years she has worked in radiation. She felt the rashes could be stress induced—not from the radiation but from all the emotional and physical stressors in my life right now. She suggested I consider postponing my NY trip to my folks for a few days.

She makes a good point. My plans were to drive to my son in Richmond and then on to NY the day after completing radiation. Waiting a few days will allow my skin, and my broken rib, a little more time to heal. It does indeed hurt to drive with the broken rib, especially turning to look over my shoulder. Every time I back up or park, it is accompanied with sharp stabs of pain.

Anyway, the doctor felt I would not likely feel any worse than I do now, and would slowly heal from this point forward. In radiation, the cancer cells are killed, but even the normal cells are damaged. They can, and will, recover, but that is a stress on the body. It is probably why fatigue is such a big issue with most people who undergo radiation. (I definitely have slowed down, and even nap now and then in these final weeks of radiation.)

I thought about what is going on in my body physically and was struck by the spiritual parallel. When we come to know Christ, our old sinful self is destroyed. We are being made new, sanctified by the transforming work of the Holy Spirit. It is not an easy process. The old self is dying, and the new self is struggling to live, to emerge. It is indeed at times exhausting, with setbacks and failures. We do not become Christ-like overnight. It is a process. The old self dies. The new self grows stronger.

We will overcome and be victorious ultimately, but it will take an entire lifetime. Perfection will not be possible until we are reunited with Christ in Heaven. Fortunately, this is where the analogy ends. My rib and skin will heal faster than it takes to reach full sanctification.

My nurse tells me that within a month, I will be good as new.

Galatians 2:20

I have been crucified with Christ. It is no longer I who live, but Christ who lives in me. And the life I now live in the flesh I live by faith in the Son of God, who loved me and gave himself for me.

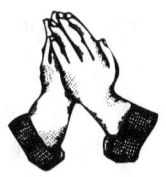

Glimmers of Hope

September 20, 2016

No mamas that we know of chose life during our time Monday on the sidewalks of the abortion center. This was disheartening as we almost always see some mamas choose life, but God was present as always, if only to weep with us. Even in the despair, God always sends glimmers of hope along the way. Always.

First, a wonderful young lady dropped off some cards with her contact info on it. She will adopt any baby, any race, any time. Mamas or fathers at the abortion center will often yell at us demanding, "Will you adopt my baby if I keep him?" I will instantly pull out the young lady's card and say, "Yes! Come let's make the call and sign the forms."

Next, another woman drove by looking for a medical facility. She was lost. When she saw us sidewalk counselors, she stopped and leaped out of her car. Her face was so impassioned that I feared I was about to be pounded into the dirt. Instead, she tearfully asked if she could pray for us and with us. She was in complete support of our mission affirming the sanctity of life in this very dark place. She was grateful that God had sent her the wrong way so she would wind up on our street and could lift us up in prayer.

She prayed fervently and for quite some time. I kept one eye open, scanning for cars that might be entering the center. I am ALL for prayer...don't get me wrong. But as our director pointed out (and I agree) we counselors already pray without ceasing in our hearts. Our job on the sidewalk is to *speak* for the babies who cannot speak for themselves. Frankly, lots of people will pray (which is critical and necessary)...but not many are willing to speak and confront the mamas who think abortion is the only answer. So I keep public prayer short, and I always step away if a car enters the parking lot to try to actively intercede for the doomed baby. I feel deeply convicted that my role there is to SPEAK.

Nonetheless, I greatly appreciated her passion and prayer. Despite her prayers and the encouragement of the adoptive woman, it was a sad day at the abortion center. It was mobbed; at least fifty babies were to die that day in that single abortion center. What was very disconcerting is we saw at least four or five moms who were visibly pregnant, at least four or five months along. The center is not supposed to do abortions after 19 weeks 6 days gestation, but those mamas looked beyond that stage of pregnancy.

"It's just a clump of cells!" one lady screamed at me yesterday.

"Does a clump of cells have a beating heart?" I asked.

She stormed away.

"I don't believe in God," another woman said to justify her abortion.

"Take God out of the equation then," I said, "Should we have the right to destroy inconvenient, innocent human life? At what logical point does the baby become human if not at *this* point in your womb? Does any society that devalues human life thrive?"

She also turned away and entered the clinic.

One couple I stopped yesterday listened to me talk for twenty minutes. Then the nurse came over and talked with them ten more. While I talked, they leafed through our literature looking at the photos of the babies at the different gestational ages. They believed in God. They knew God wouldn't approve and knew abortion was fundamentally wrong.

Then I asked, "What brought you here that made you feel abortion was your only option?"

They both shrugged.

"You don't *know*?" I asked, incredulous.

They shook their heads.

"You are about to take the life of your own child and you don't even know *why*?" I said.

Again, downcast eyes...and shrugs.

Lord, have mercy.

"Please come look at your baby on the ultrasound," I urged, "Let us tell you how we can help."

"No, I'm ok," said the woman, then told the boyfriend, "Let's go."

They drove into the abortion center lot, overflowing with cars on their appointment with death.

Today is my LAST radiation treatment. ALL the invasive, frightening cancer treatments now come to an end today. I survived. I feel great. I am so grateful! Tomorrow, I leave on my victory journey, visiting my children along the way and then my parents. Maybe I will sneak in a side-trip to cousins if my energy holds out. It has been a long, hard road from diagnosis six months ago, but God ALWAYS sends glimmers of hope along the way. Always.

<u>Jeremiah 8:6</u>

I have listened to them very carefully, but they do not speak honestly. None of them regrets the evil he has done. None of them says, "I have done wrong!" All of them persist in their own wayward course like a horse charging recklessly into battle.

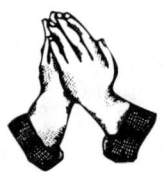

Let Go – I Will Catch You

September 21, 2016

Done! I am done with radiation treatment. One of the other patients gave me a framed painting she had done. She still has several weeks of treatment to go, but she was rejoicing with me for my grand finale. The technicians gave me a certificate which congratulated me on my "achievement".

Achievement?

I lay on a narrow steel table and let them shoot dangerous doses of radiation into my chest. *Achievement* seems a little over-the-top. Maybe *Endurance*. Certificate of *Endurance* would be more appropriate. I endured six-weeks of daily radiation, not too terribly the worse for wear. My skin is peeling in a couple of spots, but no open wounds, and not very red anymore. I took two naps over the six-week period, which was the extent of my radiation fatigue.

It seemed like there would be more fanfare and drum rolls in my head with my last treatment session. There was not. Just a vague sense of relief that it was done, and no more terrible things remain for me to achieve or to endure, at least for now on this cancer journey.

I chatted with my cousin Carol to let her know I was considering adding a side-trip on my Victory Trip North. If I have the energy, I want to visit her and my other cousins, but I told her I wanted to stay at a hotel near the beach. Could she recommend one? The ocean (all bodies of water, in fact) bring me so much peace. I need peace now. It has been a long six-months since diagnosis, much of it filled with pain, uncertainty, turmoil, and fear. Carol understood exactly what a hotel on the beach meant to me.

Get this. Not only did she recommend one near her, she instantly used points her family had accumulated for a free hotel stay and booked me at a hotel just a mile from the ocean. How blessed I am for the people I am related to!

So I leave this morning for my great Victory Trip. I *made it* through a terrifying discovery of a lump in my breast, to a more terrifying diagnosis of breast cancer, to the first surgery removing the breast, to the day after surgery having three potentially life threatening blood clots land me in the E.R., to a second surgery to reconstruct the breast, to 6-weeks of radiation with a broken rib from a bad bike accident thrown in to season the calamity...to the grand finale of six weeks of radiation yesterday. It's over. I am done.

Well, I do have nipple reconstruction and tattoo of the area to make the coloring look like a real areola...but that is child's play compared to what I have been through thus far.

I read a study on fear of pain and death by C.S. Lewis that really hit home for me. A brief excerpt highlights the salient point as I look back on the past six months:

Remember, though we struggle against things because we are afraid of them, it is often the other way round—we get afraid because we struggle. Are you struggling, resisting? Don't you think Our Lord says to you 'Peace, child, peace. Relax. Let go. Underneath are the everlasting arms. Let go, I will catch you. Do you trust me so little?'

Of course, this may not be the end. Then make it a good rehearsal.

The most calm and even joy-filled moments over the past six-months have been when I inexplicably relaxed and trusted God that even though this was decidedly NOT a journey I would have chosen to embark upon, if He deemed it necessary, then it would end in GOOD. When I struggled and railed against what was happening, I only made it worse. C.S. Lewis is exactly right. Do I trust God in all things...or only in the pleasant circumstances? If I trust him, let go, knowing He will catch me.

But for now, there is a respite. No more surgeries or invasive procedures. Oh, there is still medicine I start in two weeks and will take for the next five years, and checkup visits, and probably more tests along the way to be sure the cancer stays gone. However, all the terrible things I was certain I could not, and would not survive...I did, and they are DONE.

So here I am, about to embark on my Victory Trip. I will visit loved ones, sip wine by the ocean (which is not allowed my cousin warns me but everyone does it anyway....), go on long bike rides on new bike trails, and hike uncharted paths. I will hug my parents, my sons, my daughter, my daughter-in-law, my brother, my sister-in-law, and my cousins. Maybe an aunt or two, as well. I will see the first colors of Autumn sprinkling trees in New England, and breathe deeply (now that my broken rib is healing and I *can* breathe deeply again) of the cool air sweeping down from Heaven and across the beautiful world God made. (PS- Thank you dear hubby for continuing working so I could do this blessed victory lap.)

I will pray without ceasing. I have so much to be thankful for.

In the middle of my wonderful day yesterday, I got a text from a mom that I had counseled many weeks ago at the abortion center. She chose life *that* day, but we considered her a 'shaky save'. She told us for *now* she would not abort. She did agree to let me send her daily Bible verses. I tried to contact her a few times, but she never responded. I was pretty sure she had aborted. Nonetheless, I continued to send her daily Bible verses. If she had aborted, she would need God's comfort more than ever.

The text yesterday said, "Hi Miss Vicky. I decided to keep my baby. It's a girl. I thought you would want to know."

Hope has a way of sticking its head out of the mud and completely transforming what you were certain would never be anything but a dismal, lifeless swamp. God, though not visible, is always present, and where you *least* expect Him is often where He does His most redemptive work.

Let go, He whispers, *Trust me. I will catch you.*

1 Thessalonians 5:18

Give thanks in all circumstances; for this is the will of God in Christ Jesus for you.

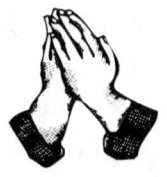

Experience, The Most Brutal of Teachers

October 4, 2016

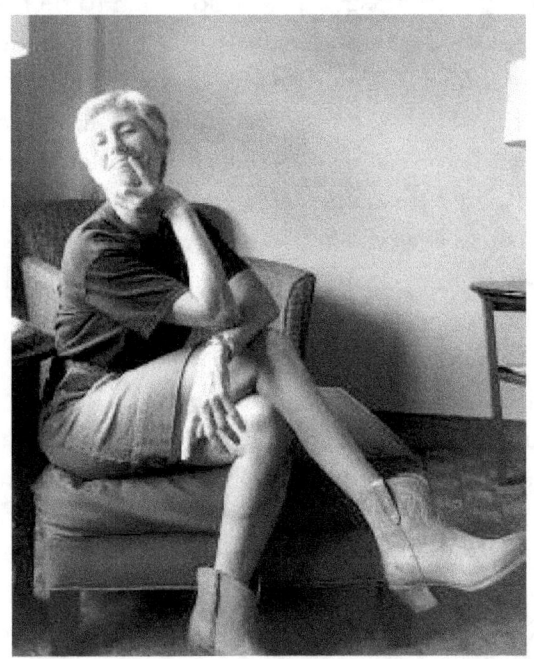

Well, I am home from my *Victory Trip*. For two weeks, I did nothing but enjoy life, wear my new cancer-kicking-cowboy-boots, visit my children, my brother and family, and my parents, who all live too far away. I walked or biked long hours each day, and spent a lot of time praying and thanking God. I didn't work on my books, market my books, or write my blog.

When I had quiet time, I read the Bible or a good novel. I walked through beautiful places, many of which brought back poignant memories of days long gone.

I did write one poem on the final day of my trip:

So many memories of years long past,

Joy mixed with sorrow for things that don't last,
Grateful eternity won't vanish so fast.

On the last morning of my exodus, I hiked ten miles through the historic and stunning little town of Lexington. I had visited that city many times when my son, Matthias and his wife both attended Washington and Lee Law School there. It is one of the most beautiful cities on earth. It is also on the Bikecentennial Bike Trail.

In 1976, my father sent me on a trip of a lifetime, crossing Virginia on my bicycle with the Bikecentennial group. I slept with the group in a little park on the outskirts of Lexington, and then biked through Lexington. The memories are vague, but were rekindled as I wandered through the cemetery, along the Maury River, and through the campuses of Virginia Military Institute and Washington and Lee University. Colorful scenes from my distant past drifted through my mind like leaves blown loose by the autumn breeze.

Slowly, over the two weeks of my trip, the seared, red skin from my radiation treatments faded to a normal color. The pain from the rib I broke five weeks ago in the stupid bicycle mishap subsided. The swelling from the two cancer operations, the broken rib, and the effects of radiation ebbed. I felt almost normal again as I lugged my suitcases back into my house yesterday.

I listened to countless sermons on the radio during the many hours driving. One struck me particularly, and I called upon the lesson of the speaker many times. We who have accepted Jesus as Lord and savior are indwelt by the Holy Spirit. The speaker described how she would specifically ask the Holy Spirit to teach and to comfort her during times of despair or confusion. The situation rarely changed, but she said more often than not, peace would descend upon her and optimism would replace dread.

During my trip, memories flooded back with each familiar city I visited; during the time spent with my oldest son, Anders, and my middle son, Matthias, and then while wandering and biking places where I had spent years being a part of the landscape. I found myself remembering not only the good, but also the bad. I reflected upon all the times I had failed, or others had failed me, and fought off tears and despair not a few times. Each time, choking back tears, I said aloud, "Comfort and guide me Holy Spirit. I cannot do this alone."

On my last day, I had lunch in a little café. There was a handwritten message on a chalkboard, by my favorite Christian author, C.S. Lewis. It said, "Experience, the most brutal of teachers. But you learn, my God, do you learn."

Yes. So true. So many treasures God sent me to ponder as I return from my trip. Experience *is* a brutal teacher, but if our hearts are open to God, we *do* learn. When we *specifically* call upon Him, He is indeed there. Each time I did so, the intensity of my sorrow vanished and was replaced with a recognition that I am loved and eternity awaits where all the sorrows and regrets of this world will evaporate. We will die to this mortal life, but God promises, something infinitely better awaits those who love and trust in Him.

In the meantime, amidst the sorrow of this world, there is also great joy. So much beauty God has spread before us like a banquet! A feast of magnificence, but it will pass away. He, on the other hand, is always there, was always there, and will always be there.

Matthew 16:25

For whoever would save his life will lose it, but whoever loses his life for my sake will find it.

Author's Note

The diagnosis of breast cancer was certainly one of the scariest, most devastating moments I ever faced. I did not know how I could possibly go through what I had no choice but to go through.

Those first days were awash in terror, despair, and denial. I could never have imagined as I reached the end of cancer treatment, I would look back on the experience with joy.

Don't get me wrong. There were many terrible moments. But I can say with complete assurance and sincerity that God sustained me supernaturally, and even brought delight in the midst of sorrow.

I write a daily blog (vickykaseorg.blogspot.com) and kept an ongoing account of what I was going through. I am so glad I did, because looking back on it now, it is mostly a blur. However, I was able to compile my experience for this book from those blog entries.

As I edited my book, I was surprised to see how many of my entries included parallel stories of my work counseling abortion-minded women. As they were so callously throwing life away, I was trying desperately to save my own. The Biblical counsel to both of us was the same. This book is a tribute to the sacred value of life.

You would not believe the strangest part of this cancer journey. When I look back, I don't remember the horror. I remember the *joy*.

That is God, through and through. He takes the worst and the ugliest parts of life, and transforms them. Sometimes He did it through the stupendous doctors He put in my path. Sometimes through the unbelievably compassionate nurses. Sometimes through selfless family members and friends. Sometimes through unexpected gifts. Sometimes through others whose struggles were much worse than mine…Always through His redemptive mercy, grace, and love.

There are too many people to thank, not only for this book, but for the journey that necessitated the book. All my doctors and nurses at Levine Cancer Institute were incredible. I owe them my life. My children, my siblings, and my husband were constantly with me. My friends poured out of the woodwork, too many to name. You all know who you are and I am so grateful for all of you.

Special gratitude to Amy, my sister, who spent so much time with me making one of the worst parts of my life also one of the most enjoyable. Only Amy could have done that! Love you, dear Sister!

I wrote this book because I am a weak and pain-adverse person. If I could endure breast cancer, anyone can. This book was written to encourage anyone facing adversity not to despair. God is with you, always, to the very end of the ages.

Other Books by Vicky Kaseorg

Listening with a Broken Ear – 2011

God Drives a Tow Truck – 2011

Tommy - a Story of Ability – 2012

Turning Points-The Life of a Milne Bay WWII Gunner – 2012

The Illustrated 23rd Psalm – 2012

The Good Parent – 2012

The Well -Trained Human – 2012

Saving a Dog – 2014

The Tower Builder – 2014

The Bark of the Covenant – 2014

Poppy- The Dirty Ditch Digging Dingo – 2015

The Paws That Bring Good News – 2015

Joe - The Horse Nobody Loved – 2015

Gidget - The Horse Formerly Known as Witch – 2015

Gidget - The Horse I Didn't Own – 2015

Gidget - The Horse That Waited For Me – 2015

Singing in the Darkness – 2016

Unlikely Friends – 2016

Unlikely Redemption – 2016

Unlikely Rescue – Spring 2017

To Connect with Vicky Kaseorg

I love to hear from readers! Your comments and feedback are a continual inspiration. Please sign up for email updates to my publications at my Facebook author or blog page.

Visit my Facebook page and "like" it for regular updates on new books/writing. I love to hear from readers!

www.facebook.com/kaseorgvicky/

Twitter: https://twitter.com/vickykaseorg

Follow me on my daily inspirational blog at vickykaseorg.blogspot.com

Stay abreast of new publications at my author page at: http://www.amazon.com/Vicky-Kaseorg/e/B006XJ2DWU

Also, reviews are critical to all authors. Please visit the site where you purchased this book to write a review. I would be very grateful for your review.

Sign up on my mailing list for new releases and specials at: http://eepurl.com/bp-EEP

The End

www.ingramcontent.com/pod-product-compliance
Lightning Source LLC
Chambersburg PA
CBHW062131280526
45788CB00001B/131